Canine and Feline
Obesity

Plaza Antonio Beltrán Martínez n° 1, planta 8 - letra I
(Centro empresarial El Trovador)
50002 Zaragoza - Spain

First printing: May 2019

This book was originally published in Spanish under the title:
Obesidad canina y felina
© 2019 Grupo Asís Biomedia, SL
ISBN Spanish edition: 978-84-17225-78-0

Translation:
Owen Howard

Illustrator:
Jacob Gragera Artal

ISBN: 978-84-17640-24-8
DL: Z 151-2019

Design, layout and printing:
Servet editorial - Grupo Asís Biomedia, SL
www.grupoasis.com
info@grupoasis.com

GRUPO asis

Servet is the publishing house of Grupo Asís

"The obese patient is too cowardly to fight

and too fat to run"

(adapted from E. Hubbard).

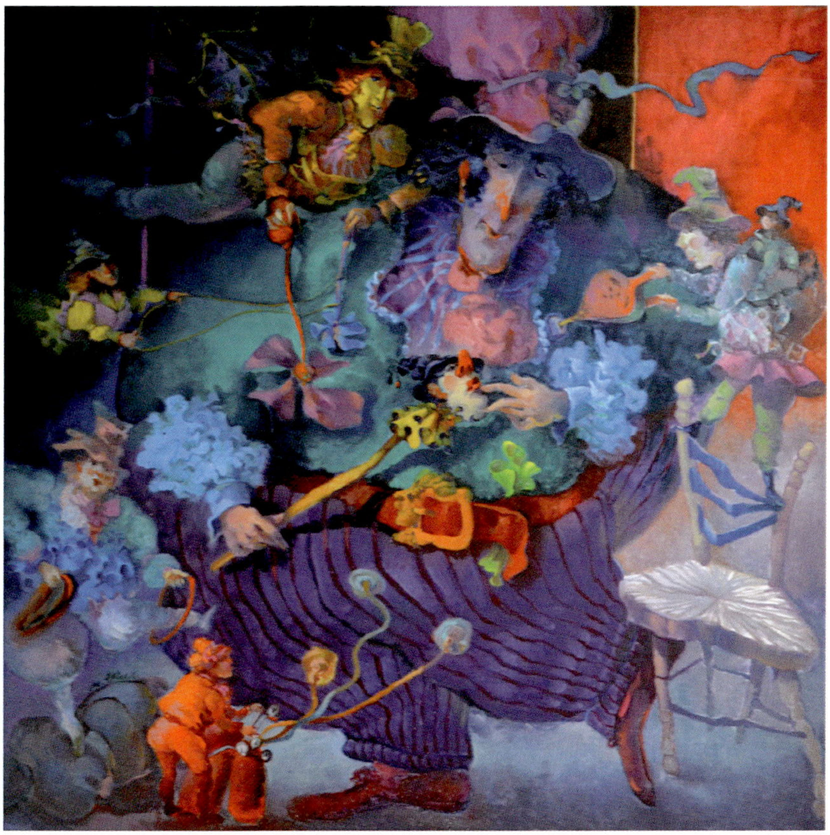

M. Elices *Maestro hinchable*.
Oil on canvas. 130×130 cm (2001).

For my daughter Olivia and her mother.

Acknowledgments

To my parents, for giving me the best that they could offer me. Thank you.

To César and Encarnación, my other parents, for your love.

To my pets: those that are still here (*Mel*, *Chisp*, *Cucuso*) and those that have passed on (*Chiska*, *Ramón*, *Cajal*, *Pich*, *Negra*, and *Noru*). For our shared moments, from which I have learned much.

To veterinary surgeons S. Miguélez Fernández and L. Parrondo Casín from the Mimos veterinary clinic (Pozuelo de Alarcón, Madrid) for their collaboration in clinical cases and for providing images.

To my dear friends Mar Sanz Luengo, Carmen Muñoz Serrano, Cristina Ortiz Díez de Tortosa, and the rest of the team from the Archives and Library of the UCM Faculty of Veterinary Medicine (Madrid). Without their participation, compilation of the bibliography would have been impossible.

To Dr. L. P. Alenza of the UCM Veterinary Teaching Hospital, for her valuable advice.

To my family, colleagues, and friends who have supported me in the most difficult times, in particular my brother-in-law Álvaro, for helping me laugh about life.

To the writing and creative team at Servet Editorial, and in particular Tatiana Blasco, for their invaluable work.

The author

Roberto Elices Mínguez

Degree and PhD in veterinary medicine from the Complutense University of Madrid (UCM). Roberto Elices Mínguez is a professor of companion and large animal nutrition at the Department of Animal Production and a veterinary clinician in the Small Animal Medicine Unit (endocrinology and obesity) of the Veterinary Teaching Hospital, Faculty of Veterinary Medicine, UCM. He also collaborates as a consultant (small animal medicine and surgery) in private centres.

His main lines of research are animal nutrition in companion animals (dogs, cats, ferrets, rabbits, etc.) and equids (horses, mules, and donkeys). He is the author of volumes I and II of the *Practical Atlas of Nutrition and Feeding in Cats and Dogs*, has written numerous articles, has directed research projects in the area of pet nutrition and feeding, and has spoken at multiple national and international congresses.

Foreword

In past centuries, food-related diseases (e.g. rickets, beriberi, pellagra) have accounted for millions of humans deaths, and some have caused considerable damage to animals, including pets. The primary nutritional disease affecting humans and pets in the 21st century is obesity, which also gives rise to many secondary conditions. It is estimated that, on average, one in three animals already has or is at risk of acquiring this disease. Worryingly, recent decades have seen a steady and rapid increase in the incidence of obesity.

These findings have led Professor Roberto Elices, an expert nutritionist and clinician, to address the problem, starting with its origins and covering its treatment and prevention. The first part of the book describes the synthesis of fats, the endocrine factors that control this process, and the influence of genetics. Next, the author focuses on internal medicine and possible dietary treatments, paying special attention to covering nutritional requirements, the possible use of pharmacological treatments, and surgical intervention. An emphasis is placed on prevention, which plays an important role in veterinary medicine, as well as the problem of relapse, which often counteracts efforts to tackle obesity. The result is a clear and complete vision of this new, often misunderstood and underestimated disease that provides a new perspective for veterinary professionals, particularly those in the early stages of their career who wish to delve into a less developed speciality.

The growing trend towards specialisation creates greater barriers between different veterinary disciplines, making interdisciplinary dialogue more difficult. As such, this book provides clear explanations of the factors implicated in obesity in cats and dogs that can be easily implemented in practice.

I have no doubt that all those who love and care for animals will benefit from this work.

Prof. Dr. Pier Paolo Mussa
University of Turin (Italy)
Veterinary surgeon specialised in animal nutrition and feeding
Diplomate of the European College of Veterinary and Comparative Nutrition

Preface

Obesity is a disease that has been described since prehistoric times (e.g. Venus de Willendorf). Hippocrates (5th century BC) recognised the relationship between obesity and sudden death and infertility, and identified the pillars of treatment: diet and exercise. By the 2nd century, Galen had already differentiated between overweight and morbid obesity and had proposed a treatment based on running and a diet of bulky, non-nutritious foods. In his book *The Canon of Medicine*, Avicenna (Ibn Sina, 900–1000 AD) described the comorbidities of obesity as well as a corresponding treatment based on four pillars.

In the 10th century, Hasday Ibn Shaprut, a Spanish Jewish surgeon residing in Cordoba, visited King Sancho I to treat his morbid obesity. His treatment was simple: he reduced the number of bulky daily meals from seven, confined the patient to bed, forced him to take long walks, sewed his lips together and forced him to drink, using a straw, an infusion of liquids (rich in salt water), vegetables, fruits, and a polypharmaceutical preparation (theriac or theriaca) that probably included opium. The diet and the resulting diarrhoea had the intended effect. The result was immediate, and the king lost 50 % of his weight in about 40 days. Thus, in Spain in the year 957 a protocol for the treatment of overweight had already been established: exercise, diet, drugs (potential precursors of orlistatin and phenylpropanolamine?), and (bariatric?) surgery. Centuries have passed and WHO data show that we are facing a 21st century pandemic that affects quality of life and increases healthcare costs. This observation is supported by studies carried out in pets, our patients.

In the early 1990s, when I began my teaching career at the Faculty of Veterinary Medicine of the UCM, I raised the possibility of incorporating nutrition and feeding of companion animals into the graduate degree curriculum. My suggestion was not received with enthusiasm, since only farm animals were viewed as important. Today, 0.03 % of the total graduate degree teaching hours in our faculty are devoted to nutrition of dogs and cats, and less than 0.03 % to overweight/obesity. A similar scenario is seen in other foreign universities. It is curious that pet feeding is an emerging global market, with an expected annual growth of 3.9–4.7 % (2018–2021), while the corresponding sector for food-producing animals has decreased by 3 % (2012–2017). Moreover, given that two out of five pets are overweight, there seems to be little consistency between university education in veterinary medicine and the reality of overweight and obesity. A protectionist environment and European legislation further hinder efforts to raise awareness about obesity and its effects on pets.

In this book we attempt to provide veterinary students and professionals with simple explanations about one of the most prevalent diseases of pets, from its origins in the growth stage to adulthood, focusing also on the yo-yo or rebound effect. The book constitutes a small contribution to the effort to increase awareness about a growing problem. It is a debt we owe our four-legged friends in return for their unconditional love.

We hope not to have to resort to the procedures of the Cordoban surgeon in order to obtain results, although we can draw a clear conclusion from his protocol: successful treatment of the obese patient, whether human, canine, or feline, depends on tenacity, sacrifice, and personal effort. This responsibility falls to pet owners and to us, veterinary surgeons.

Roberto Elices Mínguez

Table of contents

1 GENERAL ASPECTS OF OBESITY 2

Definition 2

Epidemiology 4

Factors involved in obesity 4

Veterinary team 4

Patient: breed and sex 5

The owner: energy balance and type of diet 9

Diseases associated with obesity 15

Increased anaesthetic and surgical risk in obese patients 15

2 ADIPOSE TISSUE Formation, types, dynamics, and functions 18

Composition and origin 18

Adipose tissue function 21

Endocrine regulation of energy balance 22

Neuroendocrine regulation of food consumption 30

What is the key to obesity? 33

Obesity and feline diabetes 38

3 IDENTIFICATION AND EVALUATION OF OBESE PATIENTS 40

Weight denominations and errors in calculating weight 40

Body composition, evaluation, and weight 44

Diagnostic methods in research 46

Chemical cadaver analysis 46

In vitro studies 46

In vivo studies 47

Diagnostic methods in clinical practice 50

Lumbar ultrasound 50

Morphometric measurements: biometrics 51

Body condition score (BCS) 54

Biochemical markers 56

4 COMMUNICATION WITH OWNERS 58

Introduction 58

Interaction with the owner 59

Models 61

Types of pet owners 65

5 NUTRIENTS IN WEIGHT-LOSS PROGRAMMES 68

Energy ... 69

Fat and fat-soluble nutrients ... 71

Polyunsaturated fatty acids ... 73

Vitamin E and selenium ... 74

Fibre ... 74

Protein ... 76

Carbohydrates ... 79

Dietary supplements ... 80

6 DIETARY MANAGEMENT IN WEIGHT-LOSS PROGRAMMES

Protocol 82

Introduction ... 82

How are the patient's requirements determined? ... 85

Target weight and RER ... 86

By subtracting daily mass loss from current weight ... 88

Dietary restriction based on an optimal (target) weight considering maintenance requirements ... 90

What is the patient's daily ration? ... 91

Calculation based on product label information ... 91

Calculation based on the energy content of the food ... 92

How is the recommended daily ration administered to the patient? ... 93

Monitoring progress ... 96

7 TREATMENT OF OBESITY

Workplan 98

Initial approach ... 98

Duration and cost of treatment ... 102

Food selection ... 104

Agreed rewards ... 104

Exercise and lifestyle ... 105

Pharmacological treatment of obesity ... 109

Drugs with peripheral mode of action ... 110

Central-acting drugs ... 111

Surgical treatment of obese patients ... 113

Bariatric surgery ... 113

Liposuction ... 113

8 PREVENTION OF OBESITY 118

The rebound or yo-yo effect 118

The yo-yo effect: underlying pathophysiology and factors involved 119

Preventive strategies 120

Monitoring during different stages 123

Monitoring during growth 123

Monitoring in adult patients 126

Neutered animals 127

REFERENCES 129

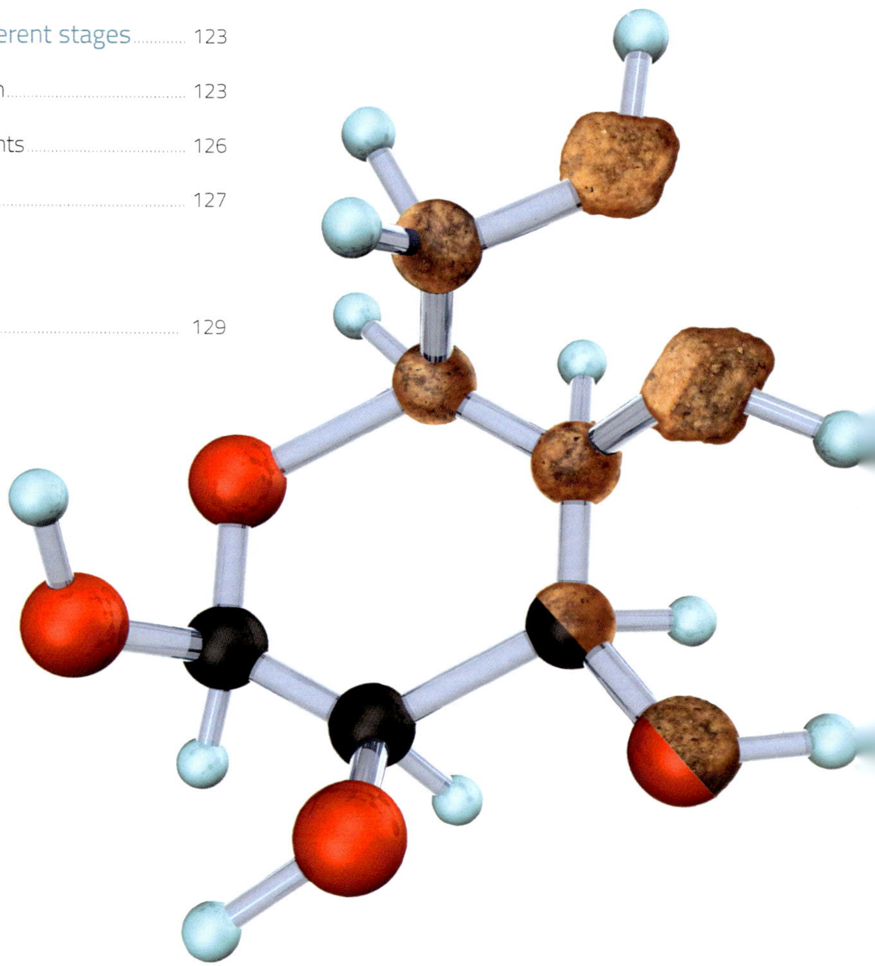

Canine and Feline Obesity

1 General aspects of obesity

DEFINITION

Obesity is a pathology characterised by the excessive accumulation of adipose tissue in the anatomical regions in which it is stored or as large local nodules, and has negative consequences on the functions of the organism. The World Health Organization (WHO) coined the term "globesity" to describe an emerging disease first identified the 1980s that has eclipsed malnutrition and constitutes a 21st century pandemic. Veterinary medicine has seen a trend similar to that observed in human medicine: in the 1960s and 1970s the prevalence of this disease was in the range of 6–12 %,[1] increasing to 22 % in the 1990s. In the last 15 years the prevalence of obesity has increased 1.6 fold (36 %).

Obesity is characterised by an increase in physiological weight: a minimum of 15 % and a maximum that is yet to be defined, but currently stands at over 40 %. Obesity is the sum of excess weight, mass, and fat.

Some professionals differentiate between overweight (up to 15 % above optimal weight), obesity, and morbid obesity (over 30 % above optimal weight). We choose not to apply these categorisations, since it can provide the owner with an excuse not to address their pet's disease. Obesity is a chronic, silent condition that requires treatment since it affects the quality of

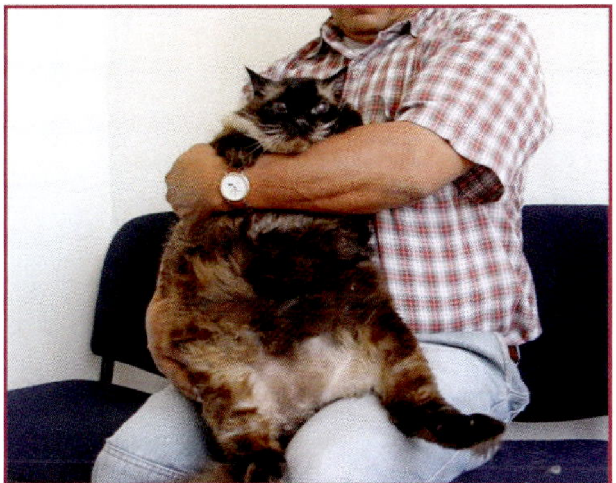

Figure 1. Obesity affects health and well-being. Social awareness of its effects should be increased.

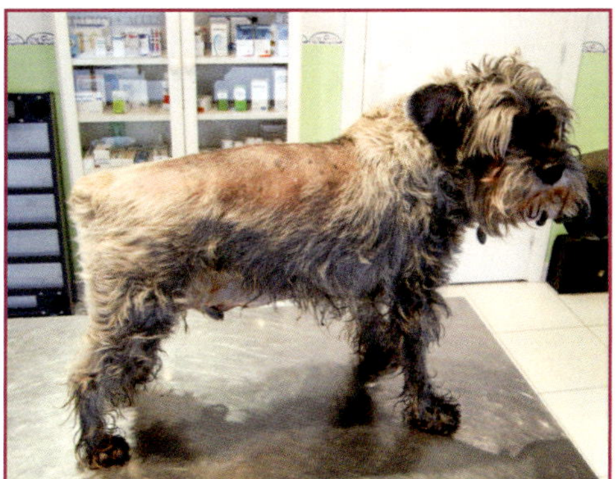

Figure 2. Dog with hyperadrenocorticism.

life and life expectancy of our pets.[2,3] Why create laws for the protection of animals (e.g. articles 6.1a, 7b of Law 4/2016 for the Protection of Companion Animals of the Community of Madrid, Spain) without recognising that this pandemic also affects our pets and constitutes a hidden form of mistreatment (Fig. 1)?

Obesity can be classified as primary or secondary. Primary obesity is the result of an energy imbalance. The obese patient, from the nutritional point of view, has a positive energy balance, resulting from an increase in energy intake, a reduction in energy expenditure, or both. In veterinary medicine, the main cause is excessive consumption of food, which is not necessarily accompanied by a reduction in exercise. While our environment may not yet be described as obesogenic,[5,6,7] we may be approaching such a situation. It is important to understand the origin of this condition in order to establish the necessary preventive or therapeutic measures.

Secondary obesity is the result of another cause:

- Illness, such as hypothyroidism, hyperadrenocorticism (Fig. 2), acromegaly, polycystic ovaries (hyperoestrogenism, hyperprolactinaemia, hyperandrogenism, or increased LH), or hypoestrogenism.
- Limitation of physical exercise: orthopaedic or cardiovascular pathologies.
- Iatrogenic factors,[7] such as the administration of progestogens, glucocorticoids, antidepressants (mirtazapine), neuroleptics (clozapine), anticonvulsants (carbamazepine, gabapentin), antidiabetics (insulin, sulfonylureas, thiazolidinediones), antihistamines (cyproheptadine), or beta-blockers (propranolol).

EPIDEMIOLOGY

Studies carried out in some developed countries have shown that the mean prevalence of obesity in dogs or cats is 37 %, with some studies reporting values as high as 60 %[8-21] (Fig. 3). In summary, this disease affects almost 2 in 5 pets between the ages of 4 and 11.

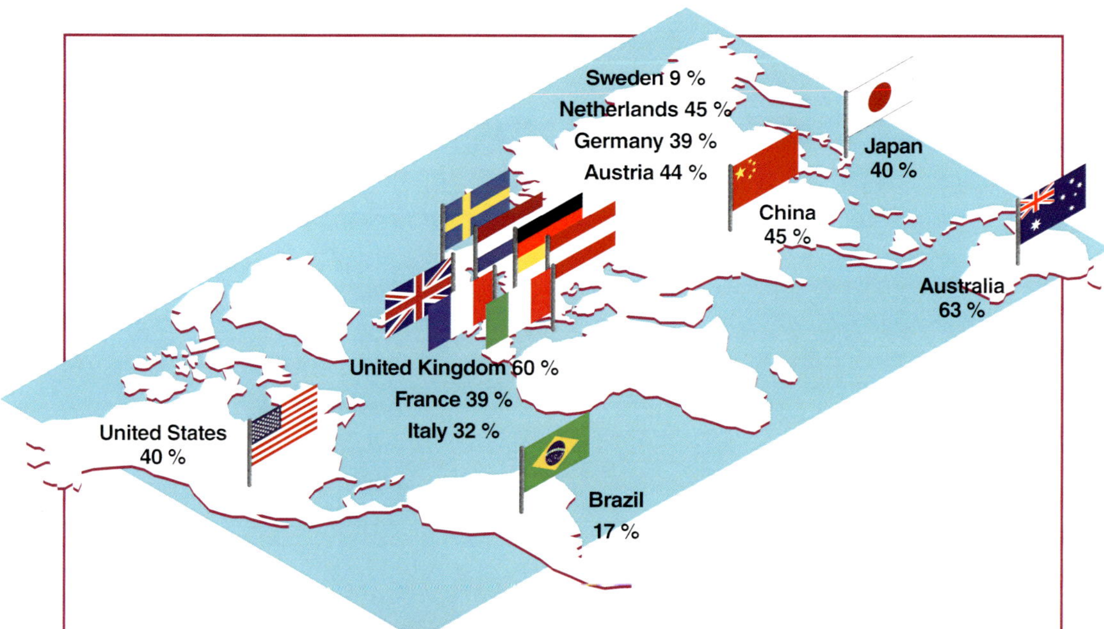

Figure 3. Results of studies of the prevalence of obesity in dogs and cats carried out in developed countries.

FACTORS INVOLVED IN OBESITY

Several factors contribute to the development of this disease. They are associated with the pet (directly or indirectly), its owners, and veterinary professionals, and are discussed in this chapter.

Veterinary team

Veterinary professionals are not exempt from liability. The nutrition and feeding of companion animals is a somewhat tedious area of veterinary medicine for many practicing clinicians, and is rarely given the necessary attention in pet health programmes. Veterinary graduate degree programmes should seek to remedy this situation.

Many owners (60 %) complain that they have not been properly informed by their veterinary surgeons about the relationship between overweight and health[16,22,23], although more than 30 % underestimate the body condition of their pet. These data contrast with those provided by clinicians: more than 60 % of veterinary surgeons have discussed overweight with their clients, but report that only 20 % of pet owners comply with the guidelines.[24] All personnel at the veterinary centre should be proactive in addressing this epidemic. It must not be ignored, no matter how frustrating this may be. Overweight can also represent a source of conflict with the pet owner: this will be discussed in the chapter on communication. Success requires close follow-up of the patient.

Patient: breed and sex

Breed

Published studies that have evaluated the prevalence of obesity suggest predisposition in some breeds. However, this putative correlation may be linked to:

- The popularity of certain dog or cat breeds at the moment the study was conducted.
- Breed standards, proposed by breeders' clubs, with a body condition score (BCS) >5/9. Studies of the prevalence of obesity in competition animals reported the following the distribution:[8,9]

	>5/9	>7/9
Dogs	18.6 %	1.1 %
Cats	45.5 %	4.5 %

These data suggest that breeders and judges have a perception of optimal body condition that differs considerably to that of veterinary professionals. There is no correlation between beauty and health. Sales strategy or animal welfare, where is the limit? The following are some examples:

>5/9 (7–8/9)	<5/9 (4/9)
Newfoundland, Bernese Mountain Dog, Bullmastiff, Golden Retriever, Labrador Retriever, Basset Hound, Carlino, Chow Chow, Bulldog, Leonberger, Chihuahua, Beagle	Great Dane, Boxer, Doberman, Schnauzer, Spaniel, Setter, Irish Wolfhound, Rhodesian Ridgeback, Greyhound, Braco

In the case of cats, it seems that larger, heavier, and longer-haired breeds tend to have a BCS >5/9: Maine Coon, Persian, Ragdoll, Burmese, or Norwegian Forest (and also the British Shorthair, despite being a short-haired breed). By contrast, short-haired breeds tend to have a BCS <5/9: Rex, Abyssinian, Sphinx, Siamese, domestic shorthair cat.[8,14] However, these results contrast with those of other authors, who reported no significant differences between breeds.[10,25]

Few studies have demonstrated a genetic predisposition to obesity.[26,27] However, several studies have linked obesity in certain breeds to body fat content and the levels of certain hormones:[28–30] the Golden Retriever, Labrador Retriever, Cocker Spaniel, Poodle, Dachshund, Beagle, and Rottweiler are mentioned in at least two of these three studies.

Further research will be required to elucidate the relationship between genetics and morphology. For example, it has been shown that three genes in the X chromosome of canids are associated with body weight, muscle mass, and backfat.[31] A genetic alteration directly linked to obesity has also been recently identified. It is a mutation in the gene that encodes proopiomelanocortin (POMC) in the Labrador and Flat Coated Retriever[26] (Fig. 4). This alteration results in reduced production of β-melanotropin and β-endorphin. The former exerts anorexigenic effects by decreasing the consumption of food: it is involved in the neuroendocrine control of appetite and satiety. The role of β-endorphin in this process is poorly understood, although it may be involved in the sensation of pleasure associated with the orosensory phase of food consumption: its absence results in hyperphagia and obesity in mice.[32]

Obesity does not distinguish between purebred animals and mixed breeds: approximately 50 % of mixed-breed dogs are obese.[15,16]

In unpublished fieldwork conducted in a municipality in the northwest of the Autonomous Community of Madrid during the 2008 anti-rabies campaign, we observed that 42.1 % of dogs with a BCS >5/9 were of mixed breed.

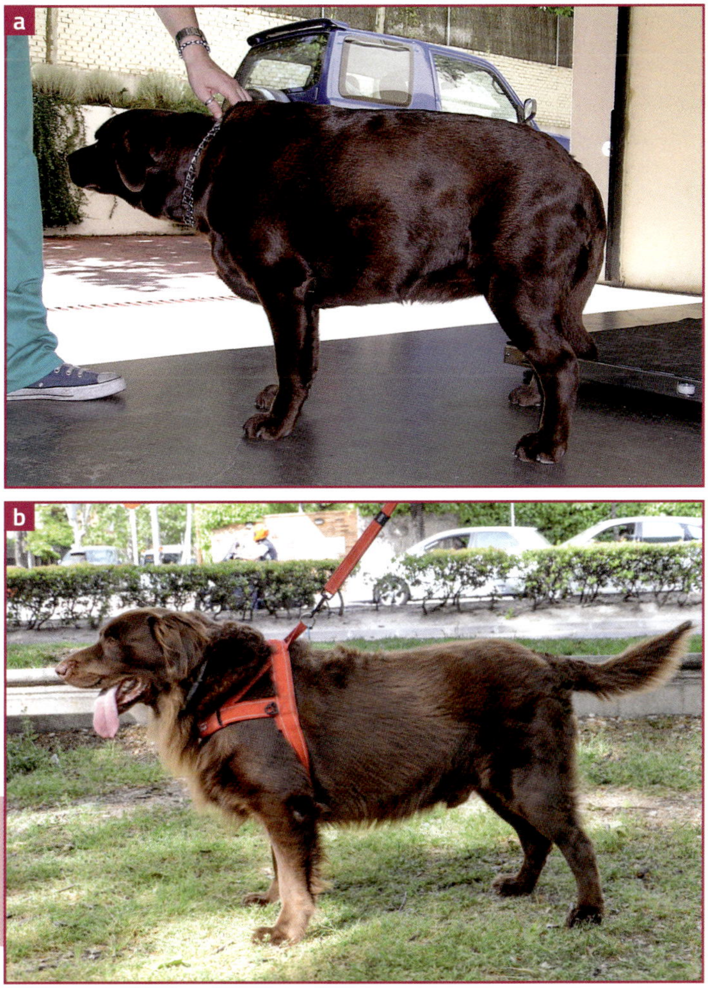

Figure 4. The Labrador Retriever (a) and Flat Coated Retriever (b) carry a genetic alteration that is directly linked to obesity.

Sex

The relationship between sex and obesity in dogs is unclear.[11,16] Some authors have reported significant correlations, describing a greater predisposition to obesity in females.[15,20] By contrast, male cats tend to have a higher BCS (>7/9) than females.[8,10,14,33]

Neutered males and females of both species show a clear predisposition to obesity: they are three times more likely to develop obesity than intact animals. Sex hormones are important regulators of metabolism, food intake, energy expenditure and, ultimately, fat deposition.

Obesity and neutering

Authors differ on the recommended age at which dogs and cats should be neutered. In general, recommendations range from 12 weeks to 8 months (mean, 5.5 months). Regardless, intervention at an early age (12–20 weeks) offers more advantages than disadvantages.[34,35] At this stage dogs and cats are in the phase of maximum growth and development (including adipose tissue development). During this period their daily requirements include maintenance and growth, and are therefore greater than those of an adult animal of comparable weight.

A second option, particularly in canids, is to neuter in adulthood: at this stage of life in healthy, non-sporting animals only maintenance requirements need be fulfilled.

Because obesity has a multifactorial aetiology, it is difficult to demonstrate a correlation between neutering and weight increase. However, obesity is influenced by certain pathophysiological changes that result in alterations in food intake and metabolism.

In cats, food consumption increases significantly after 3 days post-neutering: consumption increases by 15 % in the first week, 30 % by the fourth week, and peaks at 7 weeks at 78 % higher than that of a non-neutered cat.[36] In dogs, the increase in consumption is evident during the first 30 days post-neutering. As described in other species, these changes in consumption are a direct consequence of a reduction in the levels of circulating sex hormones.

Some studies have attempted to correlate the increase in food intake with a reduction in the satiating effect of cholecystokinin (CCK), as reported in obese women. The postprandial increase in CCK acts as a defence mechanism against overingestion. However, neutering in cats only attenuates the inhibitory effect of this intestinal hormone on food consumption.[37]

Weight changes, caused mainly by an increase in body fat, begin at 3 weeks, become significant from 7 weeks, and are highly evident by 9 months after sterilisation.[38] In cats, this weight increase stabilises upon reaching values of 28 % above the initial weight.[39]

It has been proposed that alterations in energy expenditure may account for weight gain.[40] However, the differences in resting energy expenditure expressed relative to lean mass between neutered and intact cats are not significant, and cannot alone explain the weight increases, regardless of the changes in behaviour or activity observed in neutered animals (e.g. reduced capacity to play and wander).[38,41,42]

Sex hormones modulate food consumption. The decrease in oestrogen levels, a direct consequence of removal of the ovaries and testes (which produce oestrogen via aromatase), results in disinhibition of food intake and lipogenesis.[43,44] On the other hand, endocrine control of the gonads depends on certain gonadotropins (LH and FSH), prolactin (PL),[44] gonadotropin-releasing hormone (GnRH), growth hormone (GH), and insulin-like growth factor-1 (IGF-1).[46,47]

What is the sequence of hormonal changes in a neutered patient?

- Decrease in oestrogen levels.
- The secretion of LH and IGF-1 increases from the second week after surgery and is significantly elevated by the third week. This increase in IGF-1 levels is one of the first factors involved in obesity, and has the following effects:
  - It promotes hyperplasia and hypertrophy of adipocytes.
  - It inhibits GH.
  - It is positively correlated with hyperinsulinaemia.
  - It stimulates prolactin secretion.
- Significant increases in PL occur from 8 weeks post-neutering. PL acts on the appetite by directly stimulating the leptin-melanocortin axis. In addition, chronic hyperprolactinaemia induces unwanted changes, including hyperphagia, weight gain, glucose intolerance, insulin resistance, and hyperinsulinaemia.
- As a consequence of the increase in fat mass, leptin levels increase (significant increase evident at 11 weeks).[35,48]

The owner: energy balance and type of diet

The pet owner is the primary focus in the treatment of obesity, and our "indirect" patient. In fact, some veterinary centres offer owners the option of working with a psychologist. The growing humanisation of pets has led to an altered perspective on reality: there is a disparity between treating pets as additional family members and actually fulfilling their real needs. First, owners are unaware of the neuroendocrine control of food consumption: mechanisms that associate food with pleasure can lead to begging behaviours (vocalising or stealing food from the garbage). In addition, owners may believe they understand what their pet needs without considering professional recommendations. This is a mistake. For example, the WHO reports that 50 %

of adults and 20 % of children and adolescents are overweight/obese. The figures for 2016 in Spain are alarming: 61.6 % (57.7–65.4 %) of adults and 34.1 % (28.1–40.3 %) of children and adolescents are ill[49] (Fig. 5). We are clearly doing something wrong, and yet we consider our diets to be appropriate. Following this line of thinking, some owners feed their pets using a "they-eat-what-I-eat" approach, without pausing to consider that the needs of dogs and cats differ from one another, and even more so from those of humans.

Moreover, most owners underestimate the weight and optimal body condition of their pet.[7,23,50,51] This same effect has been observed in human medicine (i.e. parents and their children).[52]

While almost 80 % of the owners say they have discussed the issue with their veterinary surgeons, obesity has increased by 14 % between 2006 and 2009.[53] The reality is that few dog and cat owners are interested in nutrition and food (including reading up on the subject or visiting their veterinary surgeon). This effect is more pronounced in owners with obese pets, who tend to have very little interest in preventive medicine.[23,50]

Here, we will analyse some owner-related factors that contribute to obesity.

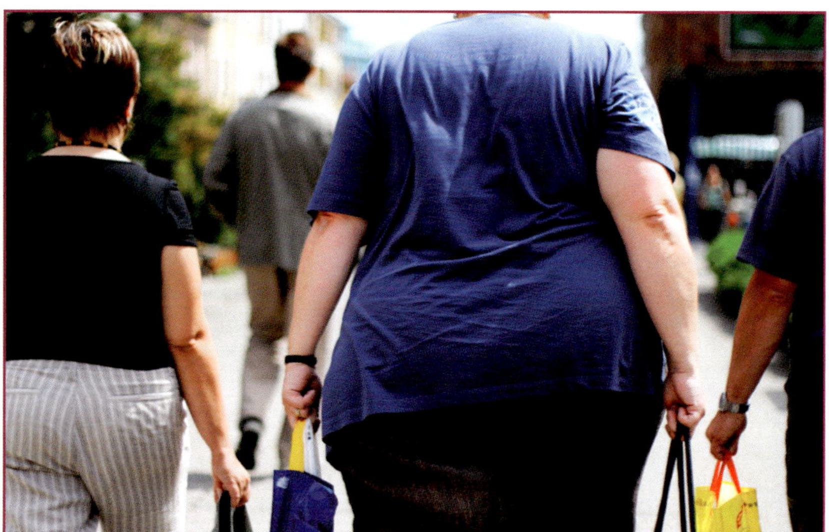

Figure 5. According to WHO data, 50 % of adults are overweight/obese (Jakub Cejpek, Shutterstock.com).

Consumption of cheap, high-energy foods

The lack of control in the pet food sector means that owners tend to select food for their pet on impulse (e.g. based on accessibility or price).[23,32,51]

One barrier to fighting obesity is the high price of hypocaloric foods for the treatment of obesity.[24]

Energy content, palatability, and price are therefore factors that influence overweight. The high-fat, highly palatable foods offered by pet food manufacturers at competitive prices are well accepted by consumers (Fig. 6).

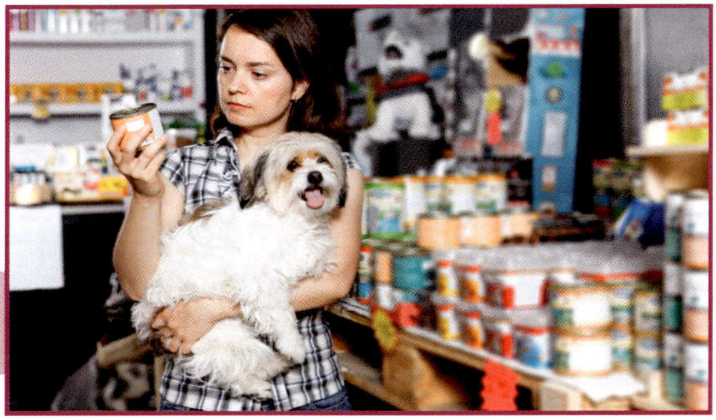

Figure 6. Pet food section of a specialised store (Iakov Filimonov, Shutterstock.com).

Significant differences have been demonstrated between the stated and the actual nutrient content of many pet food formulations, including some low-calorie prescription foods.[13,18,54–59] This can mislead owners, since different brands may not have the same energy concentration per unit of weight[51] (e.g. one could contain 348 kcal/100 g and another 472 kcal/100 g). Differences in energy density can reach 35 %.

In the specific case of cats, there may be a close relationship between commercial food and obesity.[25] The switch from a natural, low-carbohydrate diet to dry, carbohydrate-rich food has been proposed as a risk factor for the development of obesity in cats.[60,61] Furthermore, consumption is reduced when cats are provided with canned food (lower carbohydrate content and higher water content).

Cats are strict carnivores and their metabolism is not adapted to use carbohydrates as an energy source: excess carbohydrates are therefore stored as adipose tissue.[62]

Owner's lifestyle

The following aspects of the owner's lifestyle can influence overweight in pets:

- Age and family environment. There does not appear to be a clear link between these factors and overweight in pets. Some authors have suggested that the pets of owners aged 40–60 years are predisposed to overweight.[32,51] As regards the number of children in the family, the presence of a single child is considered a preventive factor, since the child will likely spend more time playing with the pet.[50] Although we have not found corroborating evidence in the literature, in our experience the presence of minors and home help are risk factors that increase the likelihood of extra food or leftovers being offered to pets.
- Obese dog/obese owner. A link between pet obesity and owner obesity has been described,[23,63] although this effect has not been observed in cats.[64] Cat owners tend to be more careful with their diet, health, and lifestyle choices, but may neglect their pet.[50]
- Free feeding. A lack of free time can mean that the animal's daily ration is not carefully controlled. Sometimes controlled ad libitum feeding is incorrectly managed, and pets are offered as much food as they can eat.[15,23,50]
- Extra homemade food and leftovers. This is one of the most clearly identified factors. Sometimes owners believe that offering extra homemade food is beneficial to the pet's diet.[11,50,51,65,66] Similarly, owners who would rather not waste leftovers feel that it is better to offer them to their dog or cat[22] (Fig. 7).
- Peer pressure. We have already mentioned how trends in breed standards can influence the body condition and weight of pets. Other influences include the opinions of members of the local dog-walking group, hairdressers, trainers, and friends, as well as information obtained via media and online[22,32] (Fig. 8). Strategies that reverse these trends will be necessary in veterinary medicine: for example, a strategy similar to the Spanish Ministry of Health's NAOS (Nutrition, Physical Activity and Prevention of Obesity) and PAOS (Food and Drink Advertisements Aimed at Minors) strategies, which target children in particular.[67]

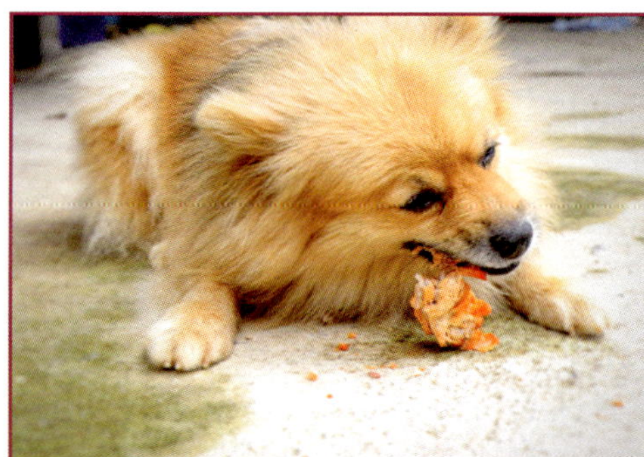

Figure 7. Offering leftover food to a dog or cat will result in extra caloric intake, which should be taken into account (e22xua_th, Shutterstock.com).

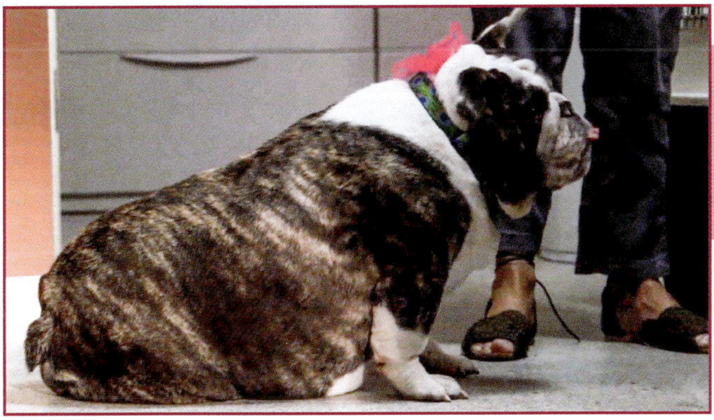

Figure 8. Television can help to alter people's assumptions regarding the ideal weight of certain breeds. Still taken from the television series *Blacklist* (Episode 5, Series 5).

Emotional charge

Our dogs and cats are like additional members of the family (humanisation). They share our beds (Fig. 9), we talk to them because they are always present (even more so than family, friends, or workmates, according to surveys), they protect us, we watch television together, and in some cases we prefer their company to that of other human beings (Fig. 10). The instinct to protect one's pet can be accentuated in the case of overweight animals.[22,50] For this reason, owners often misinterpret feeding as a symbol of love, and therefore offer food for no particular reason (i.e. not as a reward for a job well done, where it serves to positively reinforce learning), or when the pet demands our

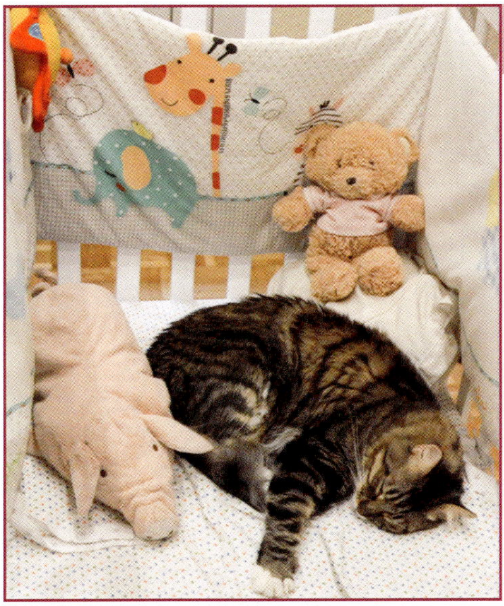

Figure 9. Many owners sleep with their pets. Cats may even be allowed to sleep in cots.

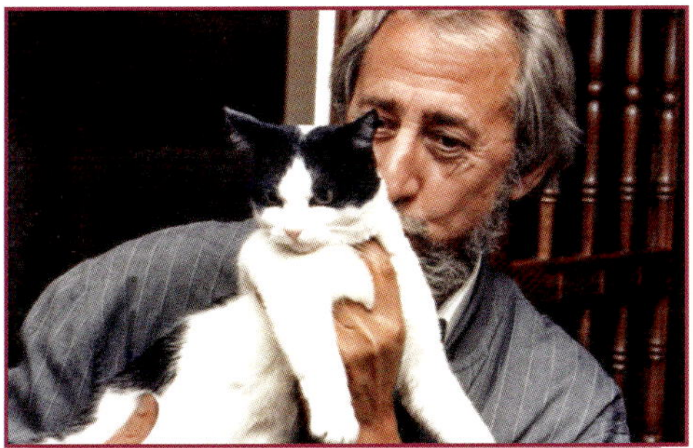

Figure 10. Many people feel more comfortable displaying affection towards an animal than towards other people.

attention. This behaviour may be linked to feelings of guilt for leaving the pet "abandoned" during the workday, meaning that the animal is then "rewarded" with food when the owner returns home.

Feeding is made into a game: we even spend time watching animals eat.

Social aspects of food

In human medicine, food is one element included in the study of social psychology. Humans relate to one another through food, which can serve empathetic, social, or professional (control) purposes.[68] The "nice" meal we prepare for others usually has a high energy content. The same is true for animals: food serves as a means to relate to our pets, and we can control them or connect with them through food.[18,23,69] For example, on the beaches of Cofete (Fuerteventura), tourists offer food in an attempt to interact with Majorero donkeys, which already have an appropriate body condition (Fig. 11). This phenomenon is well described for dogs and cats, which are offered leftover food (raw meat, fish, sausages, milk), or even celebrate certain events (birthdays, Christmas) with their owners by eating special foods (e.g. cakes, muffins, pastries), either in their homes or elsewhere (pools, spas, beaches, hotels).

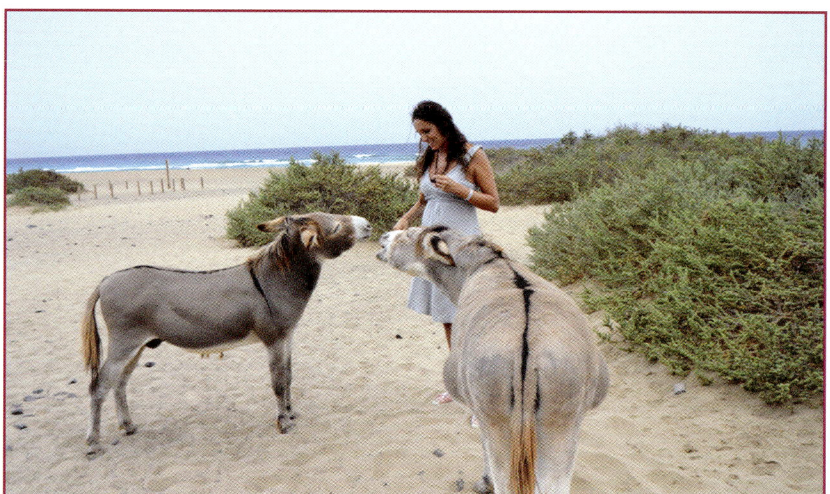

Figure 11. Tourist offering food to Majorero donkeys on the beaches of Cofete (Fuerteventura).

DISEASES ASSOCIATED WITH OBESITY

Many conditions are associated with obesity, although their prevalence differs between species. The most common are diseases of the oral cavity, orthopaedic diseases, diabetes mellitus, hepatic lipidosis (cats), endocrinopathies (dogs), and cardiopulmonary diseases.[3,13,14] These different diseases will not be explored in depth here.

Perhaps the most marked effect is a deterioration of quality of life and decreased lifespan. More than 15 years ago it was shown that a 25 % reduction in daily energy requirements in a group of Labrador dogs significantly increased mean life expectancy by 16 % (13.0 vs. 11.2 years), and resulted in a trend towards increased maximum life expectancy (14.0 vs. 12.9 years). Similarly, this reduction resulted in an optimal body condition (5/9), as compared with the significantly higher score (7/9) in the control group,significant reductions in body fat (16.8 % vs. 29.9 %), and weight (26 %), and a reduced need to prescribe palliative treatments for chronic processes.[2]

As regards quality of life, dogs with an optimal body condition are significantly more active, have more energy, and are more relaxed than obese dogs (which tend to have a sedentary lifestyle).[3]

Increased anaesthetic and surgical risk in obese patients

In addition to the above, it is interesting to examine the potential relationship between anaesthetic risk, surgical procedures, and obesity.

All surgeons are aware of the complications caused by visceral fat during abdominal surgery. This causes added stress for veterinary surgeons, risk to the animal, and conflict with the owner. Similarly, anaesthetists are less comfortable working with this type of patient.[70]

From the technical point of view, obesity causes multiple complications:

- The dosage of drugs is altered.
- Visibility of the surgical field and organs is impaired and increased slipperyness of the material and tissues increases the duration of surgery (e.g. 33 % increase in the duration of ovariectomy).[71]
- Risk of septicaemia.[72]
- Certain difficulties in the healing process:[73–75] wound dehiscence, seromas, and local infections, all due to increased dead space, greater tension on the wound edges, ischaemia, and altered platelet adhesion.

Correctly calculating the dose of a drug in an overweight patient is often difficult.[70] Calculation of the dose can be based on body surface area (m^2) ($BSA = K \times Weight^{0.67}$), especially in the case of cancer treatments. However, this depends on the patient's weight. The term *weight*, in the context of drug administration in obese patients, is a very broad concept, and may refer to current weight, optimal/ideal weight, lean weight, or adjusted weight.[77] In the absence of more conclusive studies, the use of lean weight (the difference between current weight and fat mass) or optimal weight is preferred for dose adjustment, although using the latter can result in calculation of a lower than recommended dose.[70]

The activity of a drug depends on its pharmacokinetic and pharmacodynamic properties, which can be modified by certain changes that occur in response to obesity: cardiac output, blood volume, and local blood flow. Differences in the volume of distribution have also been described: variations in the ratio of fatty to lean tissue and in plasma volume will condition the distribution and effect of drugs depending on their lipophilic or hydrophilic properties. Another change observed in obese patients is fatty degeneration of the liver: this is where drugs are metabolised via processes known as phase I (oxidation, reduction, and hydrolysis) and phase II (conjugation) metabolism. For example, biotransformation of some benzodiazepines in phase II is increased in obesity, which may explain incomplete sedation in certain obese patients. Finally, drug excretion is correlated with the rate of creatinine clearance (a reflection of glomerular filtration). Increases of up to 24 % in this parameter have been described in obese patients, in which the weight, glomerular surface, and perfusion of the liver are increased (resulting in earlier excretion of propofol, thiopental, and fentanyl, for example). Therefore, the usual predictive equations (e.g. Cockcroft–Gault) are not valid, since the relationship between muscle mass and weight is altered in obese patients. This variability has led some authors to develop specific predictive equations for creatinine clearance in obese patients (e.g. Salazar–Corcoran equation), taking weight and height, among other factors, into account.

The endocrine nature of adipose tissue, as well as the mechanical effect of abdominal, thoracic, and pericardial fat on the lungs, diaphragm, chest wall, and heart, has direct consequences on cardiorespiratory function.[78–86] Examples include:

- Decreased pulmonary compliance.
- Reduced tidal volume in some patients.
- Increased number of breaths per minute.
- Reduction of respiratory volume per minute.
- Blockade of the respiratory centre due to hypoxia.
- Decreased peak inspiratory/expiratory flow.
- Increased oxygen consumption during breathing, despite an apparent reduction when expressed per unit weight, and increased respiratory cost.
- Hypertension.
- Increased cardiac output and heart rate.
- Alterations in the right ventricular wall.

As we have seen, sedation or anaesthesia of an obese animal entails a series of risks that should be brought to the attention of the owner; these are patients in very poor health and it is important to avoid potential unpleasant situations.[87–90]

2 Adipose tissue

Formation, types, dynamics, and functions

COMPOSITION AND ORIGIN

Adipose tissue is a special type of connective tissue, 65 % of which consists of adipocytes and the remainder of a large variety of cell types (macrophages, lymphocytes, fibroblasts, endothelial cells, pericytes). This entire group of cells is targeted by a variety of autocrine, paracrine, and endocrine signals, and acts as a large living tissue that responds to these signals with endocrine, metabolic, functional, and immunological stimuli.[1]

It is important to note that the number of existing immune cells is correlated with body condition, and therefore obese patients display some degree of chronic inflammation.[2]

During the gastrulation phase of embryogenesis, the three main layers of the embryo are formed: endoderm, mesoderm, and ectoderm. From the intermediate layer or mesoderm, multiple specialised cell lines are derived, including myocytes, adipocytes, and to a lesser extent, chondrocytes. There are two types of adipocytes: white fat, or those that store energy in the form of fat; and brown fat, or those that participate in the production of heat through fat combustion.

Table 1. Main differences between white and brown fat.		
Adipocyte	**White fat**	**Brown fat**
Origin	Lateral mesoderm: vascular pericytes or Rouget cells	Paraxial mesoderm: dermomyotome
Expression of myogenic regulatory factor Myf5	Negative	Positive
Function	Store energy	Heat production
Expression of UCP (thermogenin)	No	Yes: thermogenesis not associated with tremor
Mitochondria	Few	Abundant
Triglyceride storage	Single micelle	Multiple small micelles
Location	Intra-abdominal and subcutaneous	Perirenal, interscapular, thyroid, aortic
Presence	Adult	Neonates and animals that hibernate
Percentage of body weight in humans	16 %	2–5 %

These two tissue types differ in terms of function, structure, and origin[3–5] (Table 1).

Cells that express the myogenic regulatory factor Myf5 (a protein that participates in muscle differentiation or myogenesis), as found in brown fat and myocytes, can undergo interconversion mediated by the conversion factor PRDM16. On the other hand, there is a subpopulation of cells in brown fat that does not express this factor (Myf5-negative). These cells, which are derived from pericytes (paraxial mesoderm), form what is known as beige fat (a reserve of white fat). Their differentiation depends on genetic variability and certain adrenergic stimuli.[6] Interference with these processes has been proposed as a pharmacological means of treating obesity.

Human studies have shown that adipose tissue begins to form at 14–16 weeks of gestation, at which point lipoblasts or preadipocytes can be observed. The second phase of adipose tissue formation, and differentiation thereof, occurs at week 23 of gestation and during the immediate postnatal period. Up until this point the number of fat lobules (adipocytes plus connective tissue) remains constant. Differentiation occurs at the expense of growth (hypertrophy). This second trimester of gestation is a critical phase for the future development of the obese patient.[1] There are two other periods during life when the body is sensitive to changes in adipose tissue: from the prenatal period to the first year of life; and the prepubertal period (around 9–13 years).

Marked hyperplasia and hypertrophy occur during the first year of life. In an individual of stable weight and body condition, the amount of fatty tissue remains constant during puberty, until adulthood.[7] The number of adipocytes remains virtually constant throughout the life of the individual, with a rate of renewal of approximately 10 % per year and a half-life of 10 years.[8]

In individuals with a positive energy balance, hypertrophy of the adipose tissue occurs and, if sustained over time, gives way to hyperplasia. Therefore, in the presence of an excess of energy, there is an increase of up to four fold in the initial number of adipocytes. Over time, this leads to a situation of hypercellularity. The differences between childhood and adult obesity are marked: the former is the result of hypertrophy and hyperplasia, while the latter is the result of hypertrophy alone. In adults, adipocyte number increases only when the adipocytes have reached their maximum size.[7]

The number of adipocytes established during childhood determines fat mass in adulthood. Therefore, when overweight patients lose fat mass as a result of treatment, adipocyte size, but not number, decreases.

In the absence of veterinary studies, we can assume that a similar process occurs in dogs and cats. At birth, our pets have approximately 1.3 % body fat (white fat), unlike humans, in which this figure is 16 %, with values ranging from 15 % between 2 and 6 months to almost 20 % at 10–12 months.[9,10] The prepubertal period in dogs and cats lasts from 6–10 months of age.[11]

It is very important to be aware of the dynamic changes that occur in fatty tissue and to reconsider the energy balance during growth. During the training process, which usually begins after 7 months, particular care should be taken with rewards/treats/leftovers and the provision of food as a sign of affection. During the growth stage, the brain and its neuronal circuits, including those controlling the ingestion of food, are also developing. This can favour the establishment of poorly adapted eating behaviours.

ADIPOSE TISSUE FUNCTION

The main function of adipose tissue is to participate in the energy balance and to regulate food consumption through neuroendocrine responses that maintain stability between lipogenesis and lipolysis. The opposing effects of antiadipogenic (e.g. leptin, adiponectin, resistin, interleukins 1, 6 and 11, testosterone) and proadipogenic (e.g. adipogenin, ghrelin, insulin, glucocorticoids, aldosterone, thyroid hormones, oestrogens, polyunsaturated and long-chain fatty acids) factors creates a dynamic situation whereby body fat can be deposited or lost.

When there is an excess of calories, the body accumulates triglycerides inside adipocytes. These triglycerides will be used during fasting or prolonged exercise (i.e. in situations of negative energy balance).[12] Triglyceride hydrolysis generates non-esterified fatty acids (NEFAs) and glycerol, which serve as sources of energy for different organs. This ability to rapidly mobilise NEFAs is a metabolic adaptation to a demand for energy. The balance between lipolysis and lipogenesis prevents an exaggerated increase in NEFA levels, and helps prevent lipotoxicity, insulin resistance, and lipoapoptosis, especially in muscle and liver tissue.[13]

The endocrine role of adipose tissue (adipocytes and stroma) was discovered in the last century, with the identification of leptin in 1994. It was found that adipose tissue was not merely a static tissue responsible for energy balance, but in fact served as a receptor (hypothalamus and hypophysis) and secretor of different factors known generically as cytokines (adipokines or adipocytokines), with either proinflammatory (e.g. leptin, resistin, visfatin, IL-1, IL-6, IL-8, TNF-α, MCP1) or anti-inflammatory (e.g. IL-1Ra, IL-4, IL-10, TGF-β, adiponectin) activity. Adipose tissue is a potent endocrine organ that plays an important role in regulating the central nervous system.[14,15] Without going into too much detail, it is involved in both metabolism (energy homeostasis, adipocyte differentiation, and insulin regulation) and the inflammatory process (control, protection, neoangiogenesis, and vascular inflammation). The production and secretion of these substances is altered by changes in fat mass, hence their involvement in the aetiology and comorbidity of obesity.[2]

ENDOCRINE REGULATION OF ENERGY BALANCE

Body weight and body fat remain relatively stable despite short-, medium-, and long-term variations in energy consumption. Periods of weight loss or gain are regulated by several factors. A similar regulatory mechanism is observed for carbohydrate and fat metabolism in order to prevent excess levels of either and consequent deleterious effects.

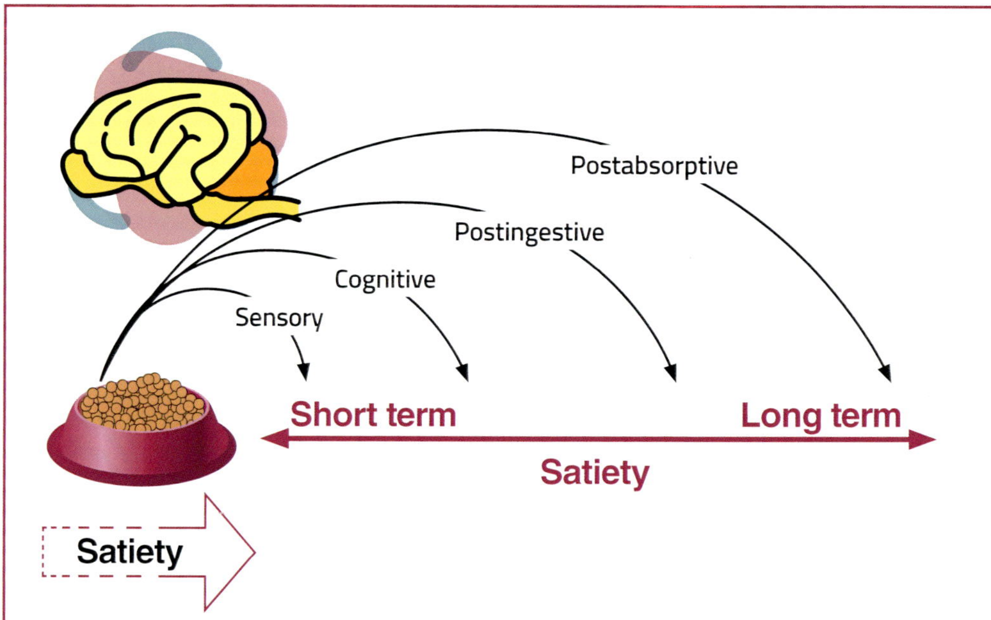

Figure 1. Control of energy homeostasis.

There are two regulatory mechanisms by which energy homeostasis is maintained (Fig. 1): short-term and long-term. Short-term regulation is the sensation of fullness, or intrameal satiety, which determines the size and duration of consumption of the ration. On the other hand, postingestive or intermeal satiety is the inhibitory process that occurs during the postprandial period and ends when the sensation of hunger reappears.[16] The signals come from the gastrointestinal system and the liver: the mechano- and chemoreceptors of the stomach, proximal small intestine, and portal vein respond to the presence of nutrients (sugars, fibre, fatty acids, ketone bodies, amino acids, and small peptides). Via the vagal route, the central nervous system is stimulated to control motility and gastric emptying.[17] A large number of hormones also participate in this process, in particular the following:

- Glucagon-like peptide type 1 (GLP-1). This incretin is secreted by the L cells of the intestine. This hormone is released in response to the ingestion of nutrients (during the cephalic phase and the intestinal phase in the ileum) and parasympathetic stimulation.[18] GLP-1 produces the sensation of satiety, decreasing hunger and hence the consumption of food. It also inhibits intestinal movements and emptying of the stomach[19-23] and influences glucose metabolism (increasing the release of and sensitivity to insulin and inhibiting glucagon) and the proliferation of pancreatic β cells.[24,25]
- Cholecystokinin (CCK). This incretin is secreted by the I cells of the duodenum and jejunum. It is the main hormone responsible for the sensation of satiety and therefore a key determinant of the duration of feeding. Its inhibition increases feeding frequency (i.e. decreases the period of satiety).[26,27]
- Oxyntomodulin. Like GLP-1, this hormone is secreted by the L cells. It inhibits food consumption by activating GLP-1 receptors.[28,29] In human medicine it has been shown to suppress hunger and ad libitum consumption without causing nausea.[30] Furthermore, it increases the energy expenditure associated with physical exercise without affecting metabolism at rest.[31] It may be used in the future to treat obesity.[32,33]
- Peptide YY (PYY). This incretin is secreted by the L cells of the ileum and colon. It slows gastric movements when poorly digested chyme arrives to the ileum and colon. It acts on the arcuate (infundibular) nucleus, decreasing appetite, the sensation of hunger, and the consumption of food in both the medium and long term.[34] In obese patients its postprandial concentration in plasma is decreased, indicating a direct relationship with food intake.[35] Inhibitors of microsomal triglyceride transfer proteins, such as dirlotapide and mitratapide, act indirectly on this hormone by increasing its circulating levels.[36]

Short-term control can affect intermeal energy consumption, but this effect is not observed beyond 48 hours (Fig. 2). Accordingly, peptide YY alone cannot account for energy balance or obesity. Its effects are nullified by long-term regulation.

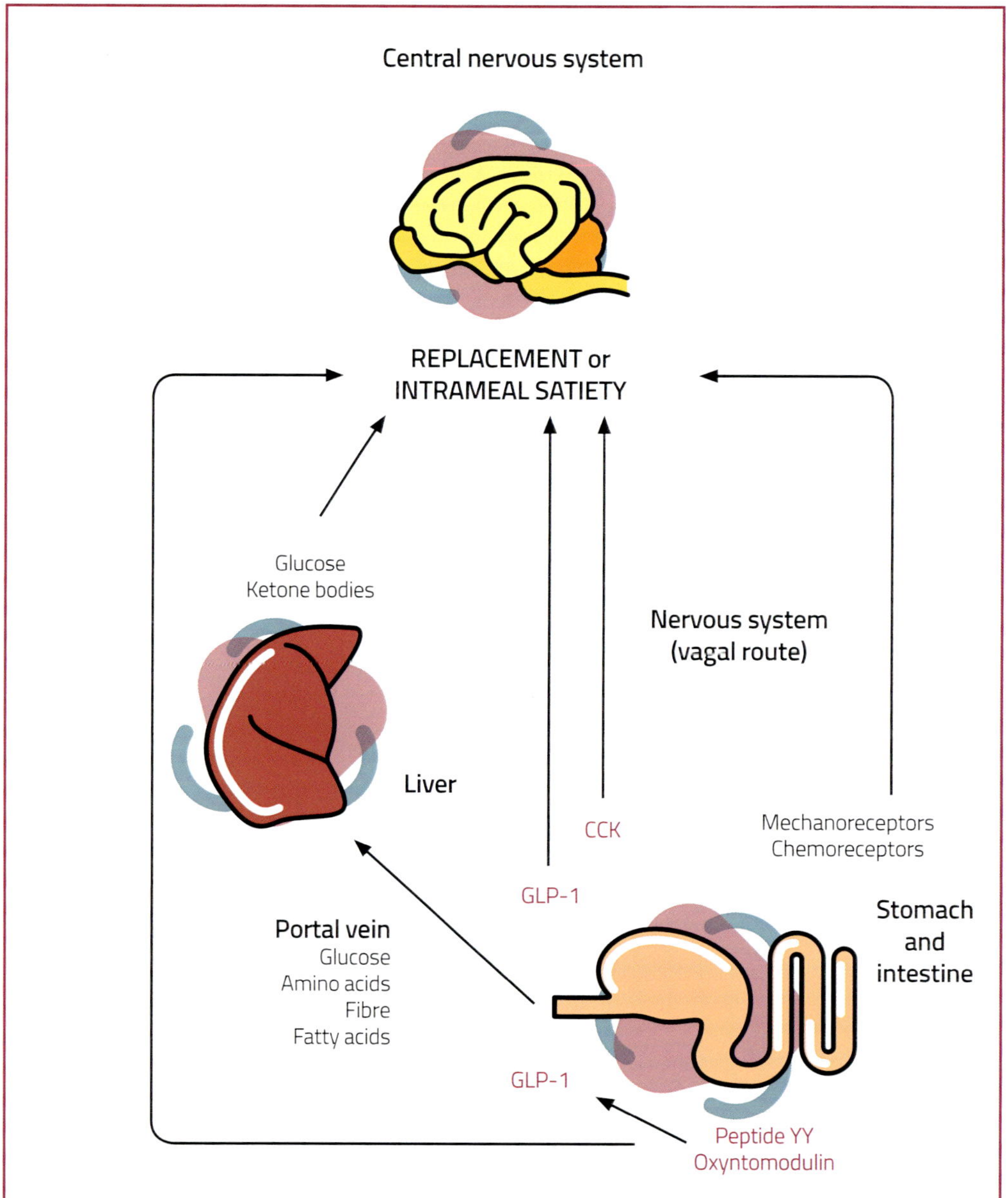

Figure 2. Short-term control of energy homeostasis.

The energy balance in the body depends on the fat reserves and the type and amount of nutrients ingested over time. Insulin and leptin are the two best-studied hormones involved in medium and long-term regulation. Both act on the arcuate nucleus of the hypothalamus, decreasing the consumption of food and increasing energy expenditure, ensuring maintenance of the energy balance and a constant body mass.[17] Insulin is secreted in response to gastric inhibitory peptide, GLP-1, glucose, and dietary amino acids (although fructose and dietary lipids do not stimulate insulin secretion).[37] Insulin also increases the oxidative metabolism of glucose in adipocytes by activating leptin production. When the energy balance is negative (e.g. during fasting) insulin secretion and leptin production decrease, resulting in low concentrations of each in the hypothalamus. In these conditions, short-term regulation mediated by CCK is ineffective: the effects of leptin in the hindbrain and hypothalamus regulate the responses to CCK in areas that control satiety. This situation results in inhibition of signals from the melanocortin (anorexigenic) system and stimulation of NPY/AgRP (orexigenic) neurons, increasing the sensation of hunger and stimulating the search for and consumption of food[38] (Fig. 3).

Several hormones participate in this process, including hormones of the hypothalamic–pituitary–adrenal axis, thyroid hormones, insulin-like growth factor 1 (IGF-1), tumour necrosis factor α (TNF-α), and interleukin 6 (IL-6). Descriptions of some of the most important players are provided below:

- **Ghrelin.** This hormone is secreted mainly in the stomach and duodenum, although secretion from other locations, including the hypothalamus, has also been described. It is an orexigenic hormone: it decreases fat oxidation, increases the sensation of hunger, and stimulates the consumption of food, in part by enhancing signalling mediated by NPY/AgRP neurons.[39,40] Its secretion is stimulated by moderate physical exercise (i.e. below the aerobic–anaerobic threshold).[41] Its concentration is reduced by the presence of nutrients in the stomach and by levels of insulin and glucose in the blood, not by the mechanoreceptors of the stomach wall, and it remains inactive for the following 2 or 3 hours. This suppressive effect is less pronounced in obese individuals versus those of optimal weight.[37,42,43] The concentration of ghrelin in circulating blood is inversely related to body weight, and closely linked to lean mass.[44] Weight-loss programmes result in increased baseline levels of ghrelin,[45] which may contribute to the "rebound effect" observed after weight loss in obese patients.

- Glucose-dependent insulinotropic peptide or gastric inhibitory polypeptide (GIP). This incretin is secreted by the K cells of the duodenum and jejunum. It is released in the presence of glucose in the oral cavity, by dietary carbohydrates, and by postprandial parasympathetic activation.[20,21] Its main function is to stimulate the secretion of insulin, and it indirectly participates in the control of satiety. However, the opposite effect has been described: infusion of GIP in healthy individuals induces a sensation of hunger.[46] Further research is required to determine the role of this hormone in energy homeostasis.

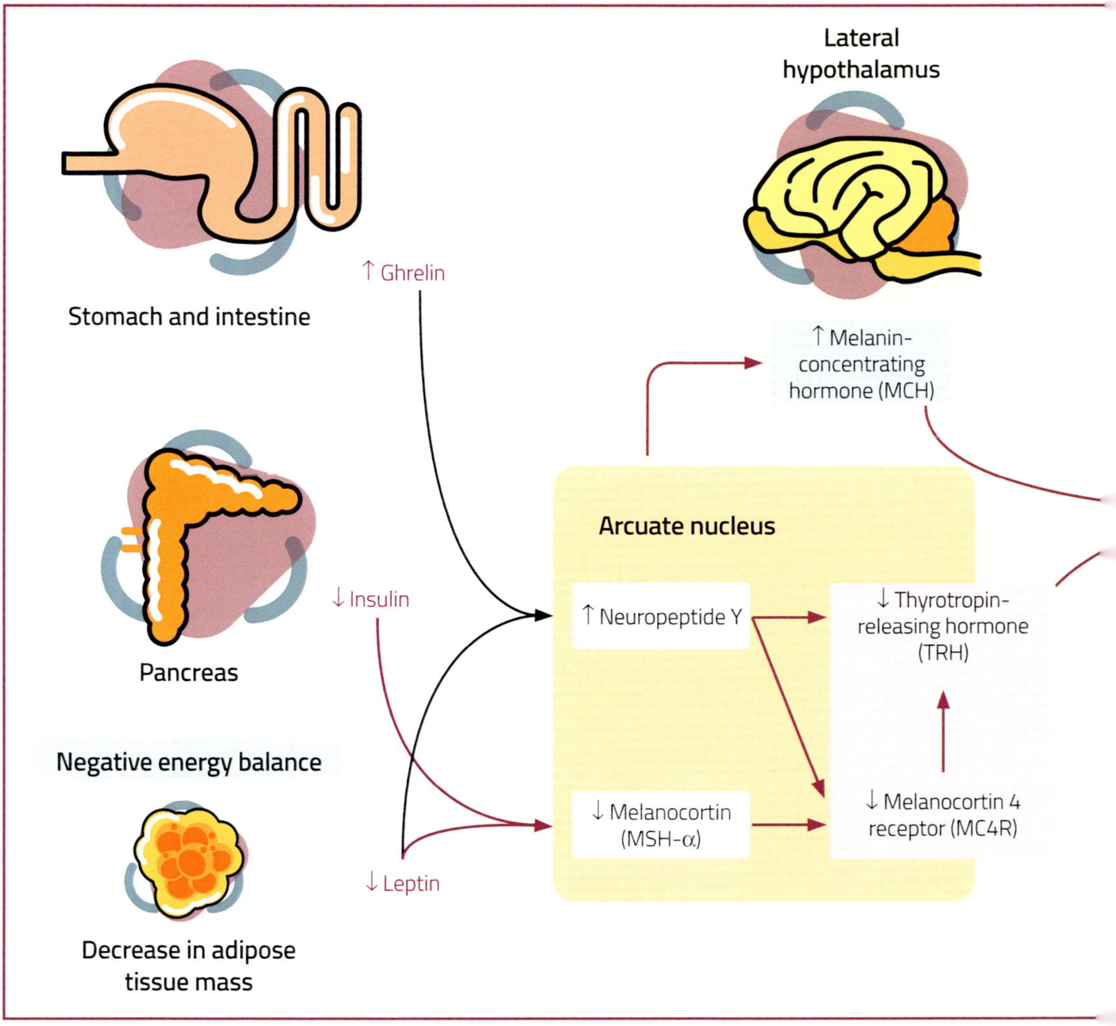

- **Adiponectin.** This peptide hormone is synthesised by adipocytes. It mediates insulin sensitivity, and constitutes the link between visceral fat and insulin resistance.[47–50] Its mechanism of action consists of attenuating the oxidation of hepatic glucose and increasing lipid oxidation in skeletal muscle and hepatocytes, resulting in reduced fat deposition.[51] Experimentally it has been shown that it reduces body weight and increases energy expenditure.[52] In contrast to the other hormones described here, its blood levels in obese patients (male, female, and neutered) are lower than those of individuals of normal weight.[53–56] Its concentration in circulating blood is

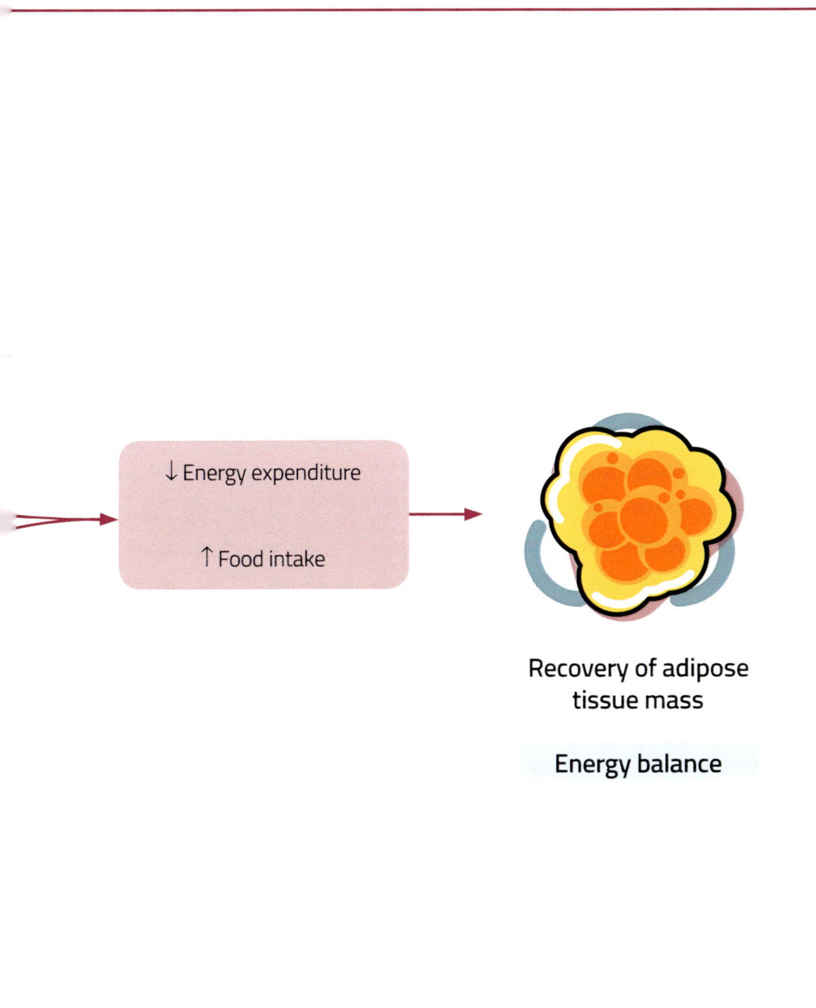

Figure 3. Neuroendocrine control of energy homeostasis.

negatively correlated with fasting insulin levels and positively correlated with insulin sensitivity: a low adiponectin level is a predictor of insulin resistance and type 2 diabetes.[51,53,57,58] In rodents the consumption of high levels of omega-3 fatty acids increases adiponectin concentrations.[59,60] Its therapeutic potential is yet to be demonstrated. Like leptin, this hormone is considered a biomarker of obesity in both dogs and cats. Table 2 shows reference values of plasma adiponectin in dogs and cats.[53,54,56]

Table 2. Plasma reference values for adiponectin in dogs and cats.

	Optimal weight	Obese
Dogs (µg/ml)	12.18 (±1.09)	6.23 (±0.8)
Cats (µg/ml)	2.4 (±0.8) 18 (±3.2)	1.5 (±0.4) 7.2 (±1.5)

- **Leptin.** This hormone is secreted by the adipocytes responsible for the control of food consumption and energy expenditure. Its synthesis is directly correlated with fat mass.[61–65] Several studies have described differences in leptin concentrations between different dog breeds, between sexes, and between neutered and intact animals.[53,66] In cats, the correlation between leptin levels and the increase in fat mass after neutering is well described.[54,67,68] The plasma leptin concentration therefore represents a biomarker of obesity in both dogs and cats. It acts on the dorsomedial nucleus of the hypothalamus by inhibiting NPY/AgRP neuronal signalling and activating signals from the melanocortin system. Leptin levels increase in parallel with body fat, thereby suppressing appetite and allowing the loss of body weight. Leptin levels are low during fasting, leading to a positive energy balance due to increased intake and reduced energy expenditure. In addition to exerting an adipostatic effect, leptin acts as a mechanism to prevent excess fat accumulation in adipocytes. It is the key to nutritional status and is implicated in the adaptive status of certain physiological systems (thyroid, ovulation, insulin, immune system, body temperature). However, in obese patients leptin resistance results in high levels of endogenous leptin.[65,69–71] The mechanisms underlying this process are being investigated. The existence of some serum proteins that block leptin receptors has been confirmed. The most active in vitro is C-reactive protein.[72] Table 3 shows reference values for plasma leptin in dogs and cats.[53,54]

Table 3. Reference values for plasma leptin in dogs and cats.		
	Optimal weight	Obese
Dogs (ng/ml)	2.69 (±1.08)	10.27 (±1.20)
Cats (ng/ml)	4.9 (±0.6)	9.8 (±2)

The diagram in Figure 4 provides an overview of the long-term control of energy homeostasis.

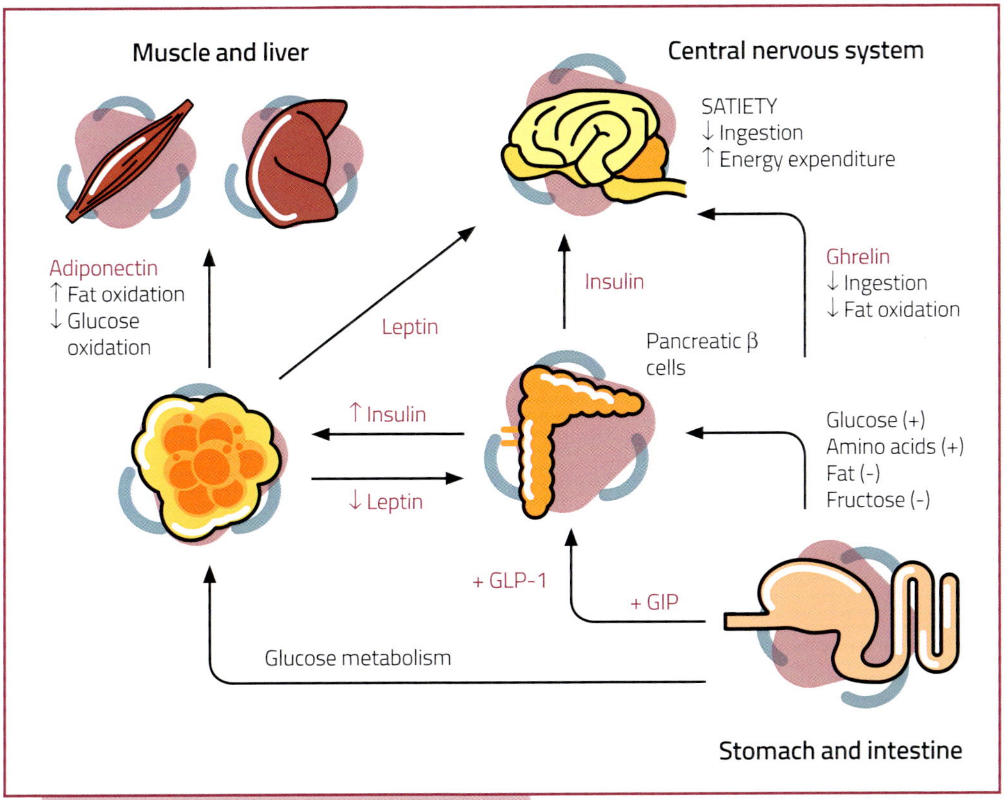

Figure 4. Long-term energy homeostasis.

NEUROENDOCRINE REGULATION OF FOOD CONSUMPTION

Several scientific studies have identified the areas of the central nervous system responsible for regulating body fat mass, food intake and, ultimately, energy homeostasis in the medium and long term. Many years ago a model was proposed to explain the different subregions of the hypothalamus containing circuits that stimulate or suppress food intake and metabolism. The ventromedial, paraventricular, and dorsomedial areas encompass the "satiety centre", while the lateral hypothalamus constitutes the "hunger centre". These two centres express leptin receptors, and therefore form part of the leptin–melanocortin axis, which is responsible for regulating energy in the organism. This axis is also activated by other hormones (e.g. ghrelin, prolactin, insulin), as well as interleukins and some nutrients (glucose and fatty acids).[73,74]

The leptin–melanocortin axis mediates long-term regulation of energy homeostasis. The arcuate nucleus plays a crucial role due to its anatomical location, which allows it to respond quickly to changes in the concentration of hormones or nutrients.[75] The arcuate nucleus contains two groups of neurons that have opposing activities but act via the same inhibitory neurotransmitter, gamma-aminobutyric acid (GABA):

- POMC (proopiomelanocortin) and CART (cocaine- and amphetamine-regulated transcript)-producing neurons, which exert anorexigenic effects. Activation of these cells by leptin stimulates satiety owing to the release of melanotropin α (MSH-α). POMC is the polypeptide precursor of several substances with biological effects: melanotropins (α, β, and γ), adrenocorticotropin (ACTH), lipotropins (LPH), and β-endorphin[76] (Fig. 5). Melanotropins α and β act at MC3 and MC4 receptors, reducing food intake and body weight.[77] β-Endorphin is thought to control the ingestion of food in the early stages of the digestive process (i.e. in response to orosensory stimuli).
- NPY (neuropeptide Y) and AgRP (Agouti-related peptide)-producing neurons, which have orexigenic effects: they stimulate consumption, reduce energy expenditure, and inhibit MSH-α. Both NPY- and AgRP-producing neurons are inhibited by leptin and stimulated by ghrelin. The increase in

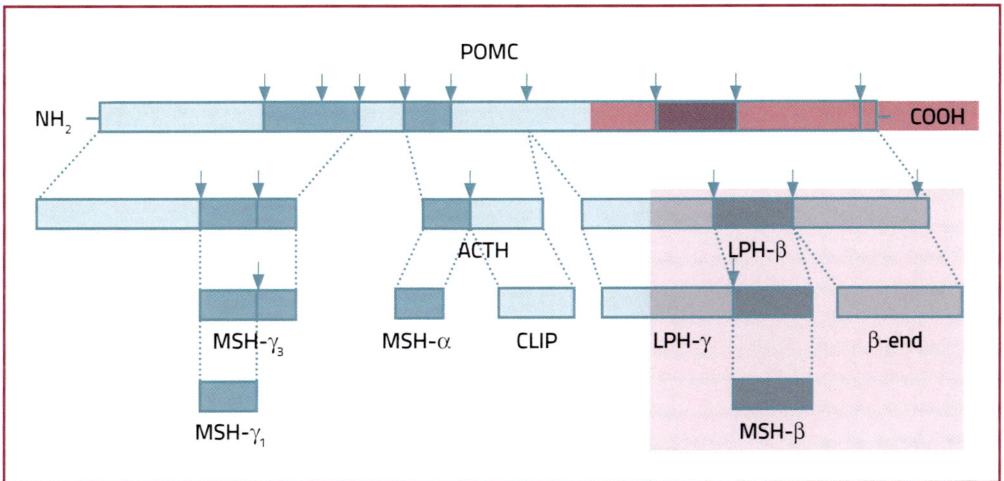

Figure 5. The polypeptide precursor of proopiomelanocortin is cleaved to form different biologically active peptides depending on tissue type and the enzymes available. CLIP, corticotropin-like intermediate peptide.

activity of these neurons caused by ghrelin influences consumption. At least three mechanisms of action are identified:

- Ghrelin increases the rate of GABA secretion in the arcuate nucleus and the activity of NPY/AgRP neurons.
- AgRP is a natural antagonist of MC3 and MC4 receptors (and therefore of MSH-α).[78]
- Due to the proximity of NPY neurons to POMC-producing neurons, there is a unidirectional effect from NPY to POMC that allows inhibition of satiety signals, favouring the selection and ingestion of food, even in the presence of an abundance of food.[79]

Both POMC and NPY-AgRP neurons are essential in the adult, but not during the growth phase, when their absence is compensated for by reorganisation of the neural circuits.[80]

The dorsomedial area of the hypothalamus is included within the so-called "satiety centre". It acts as a complement to the arcuate nucleus and receives information from it.[81] Its role is unclear, but it has been shown to participate in the secretion of glucocorticoids, and is implicated in emotion and in the motor activity of circadian rhythms,[82] including feeding schedules; in the presence of food the dorsomedial area is activated in animals with a controlled diet with a fixed schedule, but not in those with free access to food.[83]

The "hunger centre", located in the lateral hypothalamus, contains two neuronal subpopulations involved in eating behaviour (stimulating ingestion) and behaviour (arousal, learning, emotions, memory, motivation, and motor responses). Both populations are innervated by POMC and NPY terminals. One group contains orexins or hypocretins (orexins A and B or hypocretins 1 and 2) and the other melanin-concentrating hormone (MCH).[84] Fasting activates orexins, which in turn stimulate the MCH- and NPY-producing neurons (synergy), initiating consumption. MCH competes with melanotropin α (antagonism), and has little or no interaction with orexins or NPY to induce consumption, but affects energy homeostasis by suppressing thyrotropin, promoting a positive energy balance (increased consumption and reduced expenditure).[85,86] MCH thus constitutes an independent system that mediates energy regulation in the body. The activity of this hypothalamic area is regulated by a multitude of hormones, including ghrelin and leptin. The role of these hormones in emotion may account for the relationship between obesity and insomnia.[87]

Finally, the search for food is a behaviour mediated by the reward mechanisms associated with feeding. This process occurs at the level of the mesencephalon, and involves the participation of two neurotransmitters:

- Dopamine, without going into too much detail, is involved in the regulation of emotions (e.g. mood, feelings of reward/punishment), as well as motor activity.[88] Its presence is essential proper functioning of the leptin–melanocortin axis. The reward pathways have been extensively studied to determine how food acts as a natural reinforcer of ingestive behaviour.[89] Eating is directly related to the release of dopamine, the amount of which will determine the degree of pleasure experienced.[90] This may explain the difference between eating out of necessity and eating for pleasure.
- Serotonin, which acts directly on adrenocorticotropin-releasing neurons. It is associated with emotions, mood, and certain psychological parameters. Its activity at two serotonin receptors (1A and 2A) mediates the ability to inhibit food intake in general, although low concentrations inhibit the ingestion of carbohydrates more so than fats or proteins.[91] In the central nervous system serotonin causes hypophagia by inhibiting NPY and orexins and by stimulating the leptin–melanocortin axis.[92,93] Levels of this neurotransmitter are markedly decreased in obese dogs (males, females, and neutered animals).[53]

The stimulation of areas that associate food with pleasure (dorsomedial hypothalamus, mesencephalon, lateral hypothalamus, and arcuate nucleus) may explain the origin of obesity in our patients. As such, obesity is dependent on these factors, which are directly associated with the owner. Owners need to understand this link and can change the way they educate their pet.

Table 4 summarises the mechanisms of neuroendocrine control of consumption.

Table 4. Neuroendocrine control of consumption.

Action	Central	Peripheral
Orexigenic	NPY/AgRP, MCH, orexins, GABA, dopamine	Ghrelin, thyroid hormones, glucocorticoids
Anorexigenic	POMC, NRCA, serotonin	Insulin, leptin, PYY, oxyntomodulin, CCK, GIP, GLP-1, adiponectin

WHAT IS THE KEY TO OBESITY?

When an animal has a positive energy balance, the excess energy accumulates as fat in adipocytes (Fig. 6), which increase in size to the limit of their capacity, and subsequently increase in number. The "energy gap" is defined as the change in energy expended relative to the energy ingested necessary to restore the energy balance and prevent weight gain. From a theoretical point of view, this value is 5 % of daily requirements.[94] By way of example, an extra slice of ham (20 g) represents 6 % of the daily energy requirements of a 10-kg dog, and 15 % of the daily energy requirements of a 5-kg cat.[95] This is how overmass, overfat, and overweight occurs.

The vascular tissue surrounding adipocytes is among the most permeable in the organism, and can also increase its flow by up to 10 fold, as occurs after a meal.[96] However, in obese patients this does not happen. The microcirculation of adipose tissue is compromised by the increase in adipocyte size, resulting in hypoxia.[97,98] There is an inverse relationship between adipocyte size and adipocyte oxygenation.[99] Hypoxia induces the release of adipokines, which counteract this vascular dysfunction, as well as other proinflammatory factors (e.g. TNF-α, IL-6, C-reactive protein, amyloid, leptin, adiponectin), and promotes migration of monocytes to the area, alterations in glucose metabolism and transport, and an increase in the release of

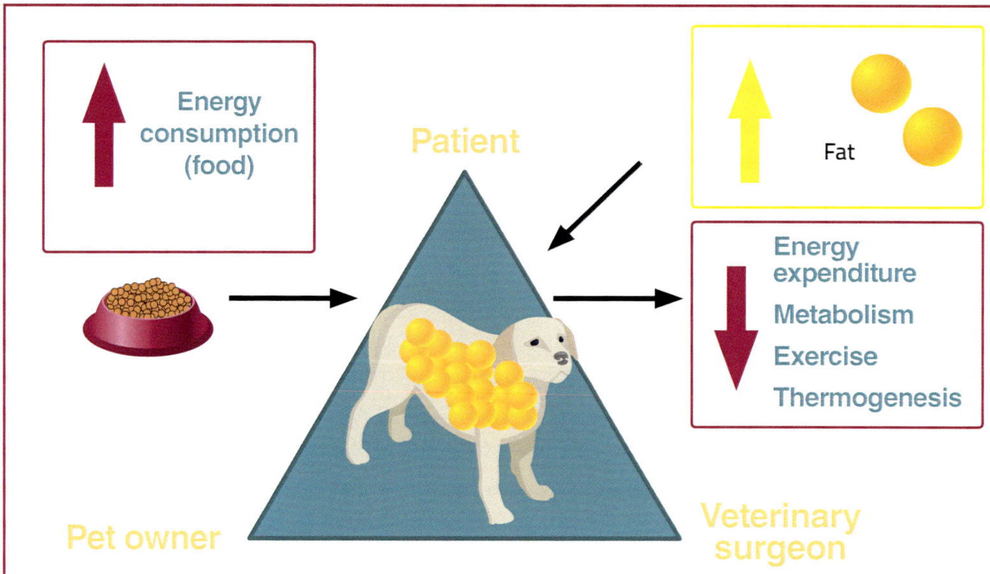

Figure 6. Factors involved in obesity in dogs and cats.

non-esterified fatty acids.[96,98,100–102] The increase in the concentration of fatty acids has important direct effects.[103–105]

The associated comorbidities constitute metabolic syndrome, also known as syndrome X or Reaven's syndrome: hypertension, hyperinsulinaemia, insulin resistance, glucose intolerance, and dyslipidaemia (Fig. 7). There have been few studies of this syndrome in pets,[49,119–122] in part owing to the differences in cardiovascular diseases, hepatopathies, and dyslipidaemias. Nonetheless, attempts have been made to establish criteria to define this syndrome in obese dogs. One such example is a BCS of over 7/9 and fulfilment of two or more of the following conditions:[120]

Triglycerides: >200 mg/dl (2.3 mmol/l)
Total cholesterol: >300 mg/dl (7.8 mmol/l)
Systolic pressure: >160 mmHg
Glycaemia: >100 mg/dl (5.6 mmol/l)
Type 2 diabetes mellitus: diagnosed

Effects of increased serum levels of fatty acids

- Cause alterations in glucose transport (GLUT-4 transport protein) and phosphorylation.
- Stimulate de novo lipogenesis and gluconeogenesis in the liver, thus increasing basal glycaemia. Unlike adipocytes, muscle and liver tissue are not specialised to store large amounts of lipids, as this would be detrimental to their cellular function (e.g. development of chronic hepatitis[106]). The liver of an obese patient can contain 2 to 3 times the normal amount of fat.[107]
- Stimulate insulin secretion, promote insulin resistance, and result in compensatory hyperinsulinism. On the other hand, insulin resistance inhibits the antilipolytic activity of insulin. This effect is very well described in cats and in type 2 diabetes mellitus: the role of leptin in feline metabolism is intimately linked to the metabolism of glucose and insulin.[108] In this species, using the hyperinsulinaemic euglycaemic clamp technique, it has been shown that for each kilogram of increased body weight insulin sensitivity decreases by 30 %.[109] In addition, insulin sensitivity decreases by more than 50 % in obese cats, an effect observed during the growth stage when the kitten is 10 % overweight.[110,111] This effect is also described in dogs that are at least 40 % overweight.[112,113]
- Alterations in thyroid hormones. In cats free T_4 is increased,[114] while in dogs conflicting alterations have been described: some authors have reported a slight increase in total T_3 and T_4,[115] while others have reported slight increases in thyrotropin (TSH) and free T_4.[116]
- Generation of oxidative stress due to an increase in reactive oxygen species. Overfeeding results in an excess of substrate available for the mitochondria, giving rise to increased electron transport, increased production of reactive oxygen species and, therefore, greater oxidative stress. In addition, the excessive storage of lipids in the endoplasmic reticulum alters protein folding, generating more reactive oxygen species. This process may explain the mitochondrial dysfunction that occurs in obese patients, independently of the cellular hypertrophy and adipose tissue type (visceral or subcutaneous).[117]
- Cause endothelial dysfunction by inhibiting nitric oxide synthase, altering certain ion channels (Na^+, K^+, and Ca^{2+}), reducing prostacyclin PGI_2 (vasodilation), and activating protein kinase C, which regulates vascular tone (vasoconstriction).[118]

One of the aspects currently being studied is the relationship between cardiovascular pathologies associated with metabolic syndrome and the production of reactive oxygen species, aldosterone, and cortisol. The production of aldosterone is directly related to the formation of reactive oxygen species and the enzymes NADPH-oxidase 1/4 (NOX-1/4), while NOX-4 affects the synthesis of cortisol by adipocytes. In obese patients these interactions are exaggerated: NOX-1/4 enzymes can increase synthesis of aldosterone and cortisol.[123] On the other hand, the excess of glucocorticoids promotes the accumulation of visceral fat and increases the density of glucocorticoid receptors in this tissue. In addition, the increased activity of the enzyme that synthesises glucocorticoids (11β-hydroxysteroid-dehydrogenase type 1) contributes to the accumulation of visceral fat by promoting adipocyte hypertrophy and increased activity of lipoprotein lipase.[125] Vitamin D_3 (calcitriol) has been recently implicated in this process, although further studies are required to fully understand its role.[125]

Regarding the onset of inflammation in the context of obesity, it is not clear whether high levels of proinflammatory factors serve as indicators of a systemic inflammatory process or are simply a reflection of the bioactive molecules released in response to hypoxia.[50] High levels of expression of hypoxia-inducible factor 1α (HIF-1α), an indicator of a lack of tissue oxygenation, appear to play a fundamental role in this process. HIF-1α triggers the production and release of inflammatory cytokines, thus underscoring the key role of hypoxic conditions in the inflammatory cascade.[98,126]

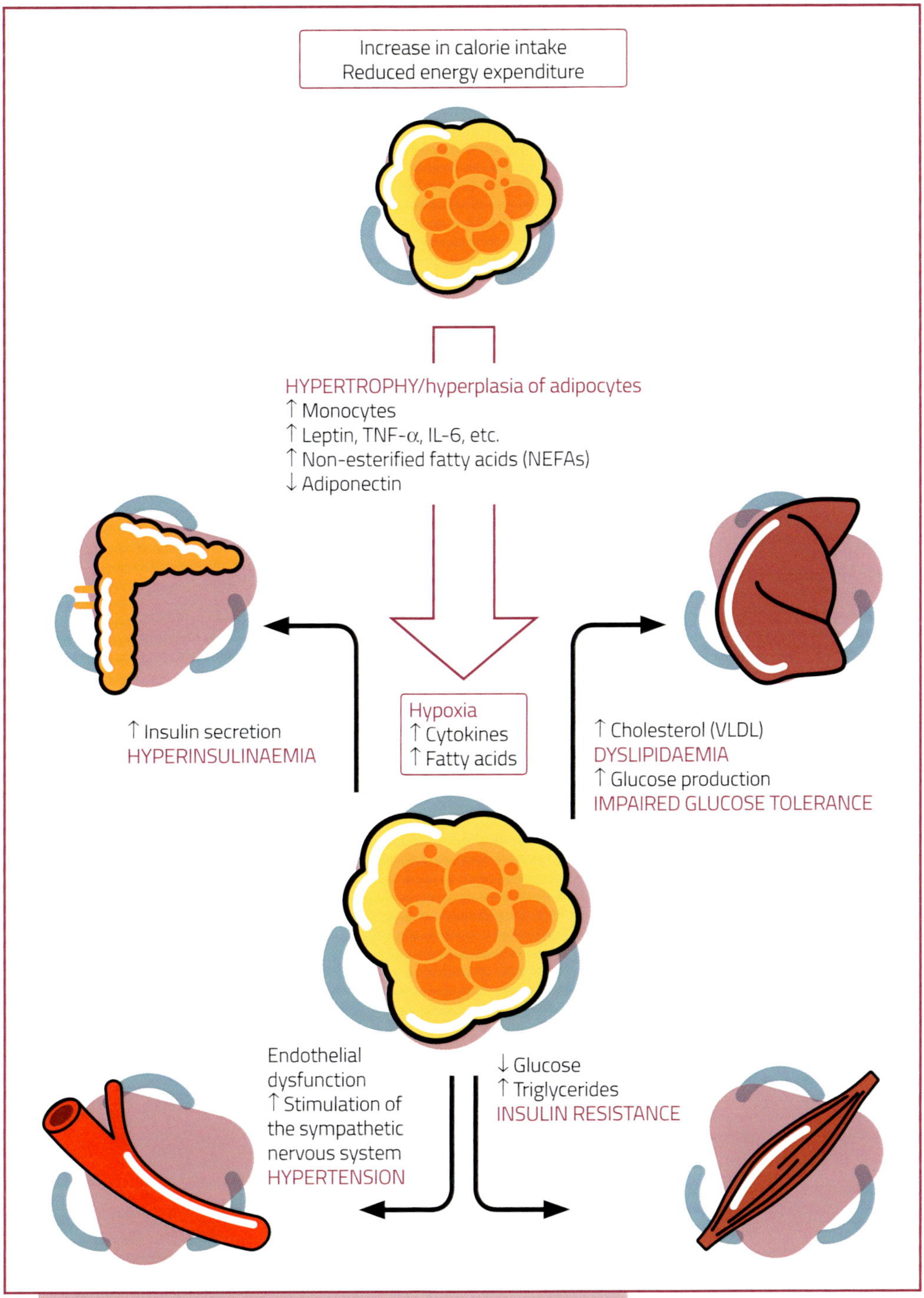

Figure 7. Comorbidities associated with metabolic syndrome (X or Reaven's syndrome) resulting from obesity.

OBESITY AND FELINE DIABETES

Feline diabetes mellitus is an endocrine disease that affects 1 in 200 cats. Prevalence ranges from 0.21 % in Sweden to 1.24 % in the United States.[127–129] In most cases it resembles human type 2 diabetes, in which the combination of environmental and genetic factors leads to deterioration of the pancreas and insulin resistance. Obesity has been proposed as one of the factors involved.[130] However, a mean prevalence of obesity in cats of 38 % suggests that this disease has a genetic component. In human medicine over 70 genes have been involved, while in common cats 2 genes have been identified.[131,132] Some breeds, including the Norwegian Forest and Burmese, appear to be predisposed to the development of diabetes, although this hypothesis is controversial and findings vary depending on geographical location. These same breeds display a tendency to develop overweight. More research is needed to elucidate the genetic basis of feline diabetes.

In addition to insulin, another hormone synthesised in the pancreatic β cells is involved in the control of satiety: amylin. Both hormones are secreted simultaneously. Amylin participates in the regulation of energy in the short and long term: it decreases consumption, decreases gastric emptying, controls (inhibits) glucagon secretion, and increases energy expenditure. While the underlying mechanism is unclear, an association with the expression of thermogenin or UCP1 has been proposed.[133] Amylin acts by stimulating specific receptors in the brainstem and cerebellum that transmit signals to the arcuate nucleus and the ventromedial hypothalamus and stop food consumption (i.e. promote satiety). It is a physiological regulator of ration size, since its effects are dose-dependent. On the other hand, as described for leptin, the plasma concentration of amylin increases with fat deposition, decreasing body weight and overfat. More studies are required to understand the underlying mechanism.

What happens in obese cats?[134,135] This is explained in Figure 8. We have already discussed the effect of fatty acids on adipokines and their role in insulin resistance, hyperglycaemia, inhibition of glucose metabolism, and hyperinsulinism.[130,136,137] One compensatory response to hyperglycaemia is an increase in the secretion of GLP-1, which in turn increases the synthesis and release of insulin, resulting in the exhaustion of pancreatic β cells. Hyperinsulinism is accompanied by a simultaneous increase in the secretion of amylin. If this situation persists, the pancreatic glandular tissue is replaced with intra- or extracellular amyloid tissue, resulting in degeneration of the pancreas, which further promotes hyperglycaemia, emptying of the stomach, and very high levels of glucagon secretion.

Prevention of this process, as described above, is based on the control of feeding and overweight in cats.

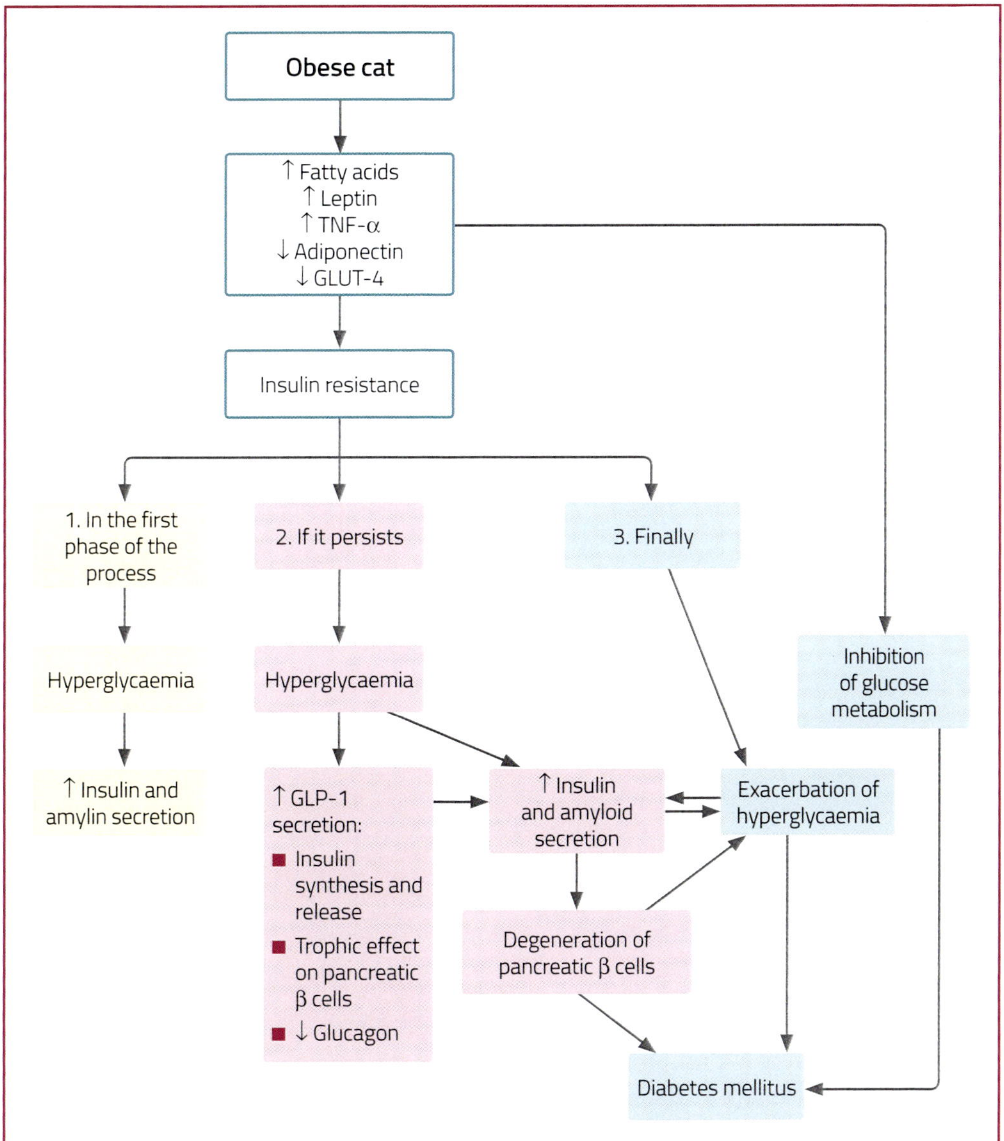

Figure 8. Diagram outlining the pathogenesis of diabetes mellitus in obese cats.

3 Identification and evaluation of obese patients

WEIGHT DENOMINATIONS AND ERRORS IN CALCULATING WEIGHT

In any weight-loss programme it is necessary to establish the degree of overweight (overfat) and the target weight of the patient, as these will have a direct bearing on the animal's nutritional requirements. However, this parameter per se is of little use to evaluate changes in body composition. We must determine the relationship between overfat and overmass (or overweight).

A patient that maintains optimal weight and body composition throughout their life will have a longer life expectancy and better quality of life.[1,2] As such, optimal weight is an indicator of health. It should be borne in mind that variations in weight are the first indicators of potential disease. Table 1 can serve as a useful guide.

Table 1. Weight alterations as an indicator of disease.

Status	Weight variation	Period
Healthy	2–3.5 %	1–3 months
Suspected disease	5 %	6 months
Disease	>10 %	<6 months

Throughout this book we will use the terms **ideal, optimal, and recommended** weight: all are synonyms for the weight that corresponds to a given animal's size (stature) and body composition. **Target weight** will be used when referring to specific programmes for the control of obesity: this is the weight that should initially be reached, and may then be modified during treatment. **Current weight** corresponds to the weight of the pet at a given time and is not necessarily the same as optimal weight.

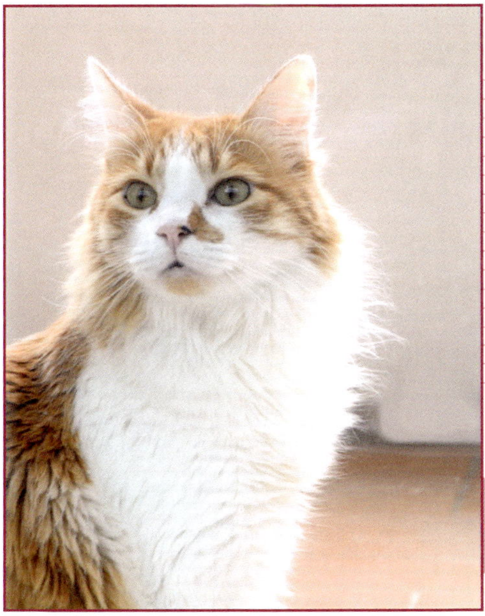

Traditionally, veterinary surgeons and those working with pets have used breed standards when evaluating dogs and cats. However, we have forgotten to consider body condition.

Figure 1. Evaluation in cats is less complicated since there are no major weight differences between breeds.

The designated weight for a given breed and sex will involve some degree of error, particularly in dogs, for which over 400 recognised breeds are described. The situation is less complicated in cats; all breeds have similar geometry and there are no major differences in weight between breeds (Fig. 1).

The first type of error is due to the fact that the calculation used may not be based on objective parameters: breed conformation is determined by market rules and the particular interests of breeders, clubs, or federations. As with advertisements for infant formulas, overweight pets are associated with a better image and considered more "healthy", particularly Molosser dog breeds. The World Canine Organization and the Kennel Club do not establish weights for specific breeds, stating only that breeds of excessive weight are excluded. The same applies to cats (Fédération Internationale Féline). Orientative weight tables published in recognised veterinary medicine publications can differ by up to 25–30 % in terms of the weight intervals stated for a given breed and sex. For example, a male Samoyed can weigh 20–30 kg (50 %) or 20–27 kg (35 %).

Example

Male Labrador, aged 9 years, with a current weight of 40.6 kg and hip arthropathy (Fig. 2). What is this dog's ideal weight?

According to the breed standard, it is 29.5–36 kg (i.e. there is a range of 6.5 kg or a variation of 22 %). Based on these two values, the animal would have an overweight of 38 % and 13 %, respectively.

We would assign this dog a BCS of 8/9, overweight of 25–30 %, and an optimal weight of 31 kg, values that differ significantly to those provided using prediction tables.

As is clear, this system to establish the optimal weight lacks professional validity.

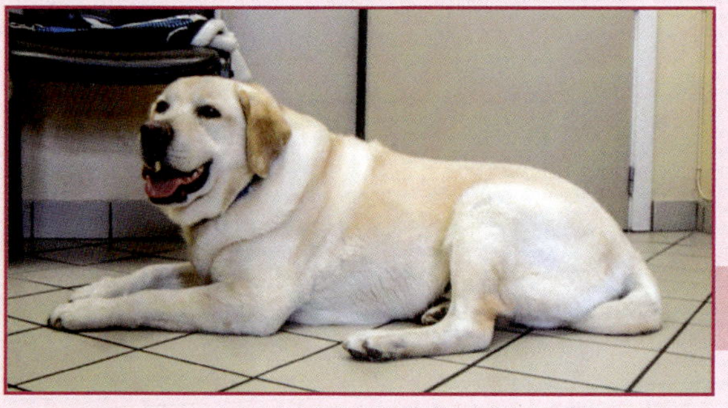

Figure 2. Male Labrador Retriever with a current weight of 40.6 kg.

On the other hand, the use of breed standards is limiting in the case of mixed-breed patients. What is the optimal weight? In some cases a certain phenotype predominates, but others can be more complicated (Fig. 3).

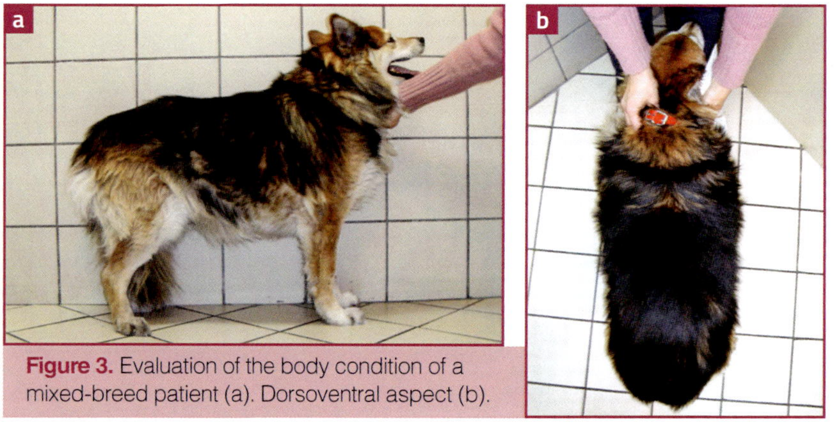

Figure 3. Evaluation of the body condition of a mixed-breed patient (a). Dorsoventral aspect (b).

Finally, in addition to its importance in relation to nutrition and feeding of dogs and cats, knowing how to determine an animal's optimal weight can help us save on management costs and, in some cases, to work within the limits of safety. This concept is explained below using an example.

Example

Tosca is a 7-year-old Bulldog with a weight of 27.6 kg and a BCS of 8/9 (Fig. 4). She is brought to the clinic for an ovariohysterectomy. The estimated duration of the surgery is 30 minutes. According to the attached table, the cost of this procedure would be 20 % less if *Tosca* was of optimal weight.

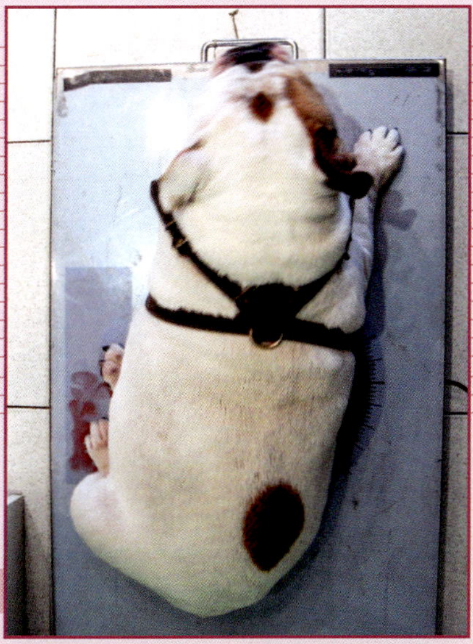

Figure 4. Appearance of the patient.

Weight		Induction		Maintenance		Cost of induction + maintenance
		Dose	Volume	Dose	Volume	
		(3 mg/kg)	(10 mg/ml)	(0.3 mg/kg/min)	(10 mg/ml)	(0.45/ml)
Actual	27.6 kg	82.8 mg	8.28 ml	248.4 mg	24.84 ml	€14.9
Optimal	21.2 kg	63.6 mg	6.36 ml	190.8 mg	19.08 ml	€11.4

BODY COMPOSITION, EVALUATION, AND WEIGHT

The weight (mass) of healthy, adult pets is the sum of the mass of the proportions of each of the major tissue types, which should remain stable throughout life. Fat is the only tissue that continues to be deposited once growth is completed. Therefore, the energy content of the organism follows an exponential or J-shaped curve (Fig. 5), similar to that depicting fat content. From the point of view of body composition, growth ends and the adult (maintenance) stage begins when every unit of weight gained (expressed in dry matter) consists exclusively of fat. For this reason it is important to determine body composition.

In adult dogs lean tissue (protein, glycogen, phospholipids, and ashes) accounts for approximately 80 % of body mass, and fat accounts for about 20 %.

In general, there are three known intrinsic factors that define adipose tissue content: species,[3] breed,[4–6] and sex.[4,5,7–11] As a rule, dogs with an ideal conformation have a fat content of 19 %[5,7,12,13,14] (i.e. an 80:20 lean tissue to fat mass ratio), while in cats this value is 29 %[8,14–16] (i.e. a ratio of 70:30).

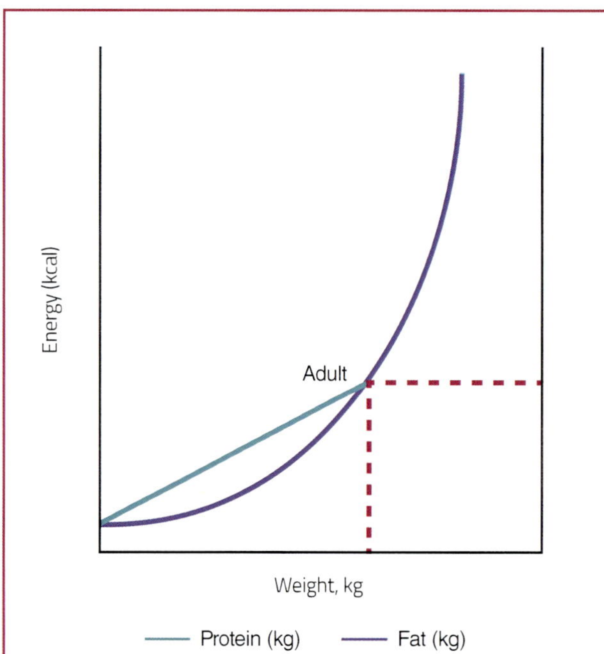

Figure 5. Exponential growth curve depicting the energy content of an organism.

Breed predisposition to obesity was already described over 30 years ago.[17,18] One study demonstrated differences in the body composition of dog breeds of different genetic origins, sizes, and morphometric characteristics.[4] Evaluation of six pure breeds showed that the Greyhounds had the lowest levels of body fat (8 %), while the Siberian Husky and Rottweiler breeds had the highest (31 %). In the middle range (22–25 %) were the Poodle, Golden Retriever, and Dachshund (Fig. 6). The differences in body composition are justified by selection according to aptitude, as previously demonstrated.[19]

Owing to the small number of studies performed and the small sample sizes involved, there are no conclusive data demonstrating a correlation between body composition and sex. In general, body fat content appears to be about 25 % higher in females than males (Fig. 7). These data are in line with precedents established based on observations made in livestock and in human medicine.[20]

In both cases, the differences are not statistically significant, but should be borne in mind when establishing maintenance energy requirements.

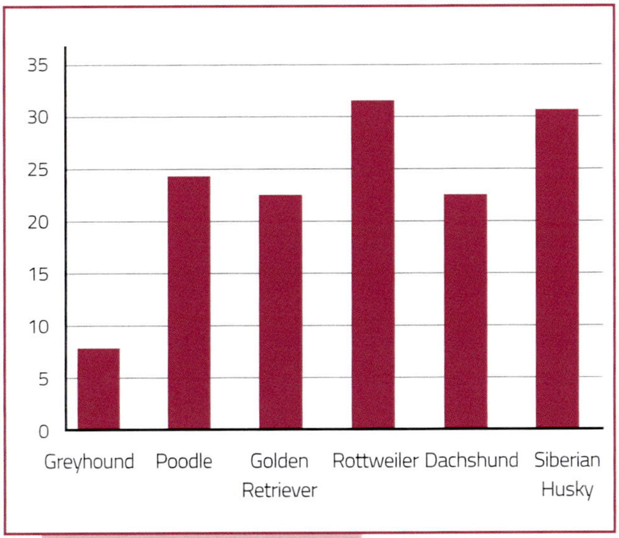

Figure 6. Percentage body fat in different dog breeds.

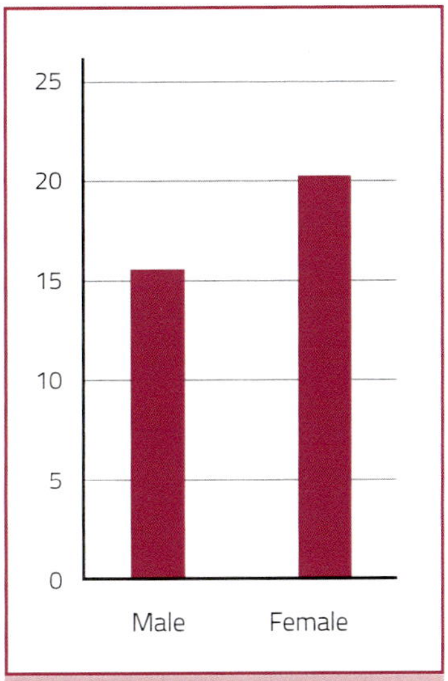

Figure 7. Body fat content of males and females.

DIAGNOSTIC METHODS IN RESEARCH

Chemical cadaver analysis

This technique is based on the dissection of organs and tissues of animal cadavers for chemical analysis in the laboratory.[3,15,21,22] The brain, heart, intestines, and other organs (up to a total of 21 tissue types) are removed. Dissection usually takes over 4 hours and is performed by several technicians. Once the tissues are obtained, they are dried at low temperatures for 15 days until they reach a constant weight. Water accounts for the difference in weight between fresh and dried samples. The tissues are subsequently freeze-dried. Next, the proportions of the major components (lean tissue, fat, and bone) are determined in accordance with the protocols of the Association of Analytical Communities (AOAC International).[54]

In vitro studies

Heavy isotopes: deuterium oxide

The technique is based on the concentration of water in lean tissue (73.2 %) and its rate of disappearance, from which the proportion of lean mass is calculated. Deuterium oxide (D_2O), which has a low level of toxicity at low doses (275 mg/kg), is used for this purpose. Plasma samples are obtained at different time points and the concentration of D_2O and the total percentage of water are determined. The results obtained using equations to predict body composition correlate well with chemical composition findings. Fat content is calculated based on the difference between the two values.

This method has been used in canids and in the field of research.[23–26] The two main problems with this technique are the lack of homogeneity in the amount of adipose tissue between thin and obese animals, and the fact that the hydration of lean tissue also differs between animals with different body conditions. Nonetheless, it is the reference method for all other techniques. It has certain limitations from the practical point of view: it requires expensive equipment, requires anaesthesia of the patient, cannot be repeated until after 7 days, and can suffer from inherent calculation errors (since it does not differentiate between water in bone tissue and water in muscle).

In vivo studies

Dual-energy X-ray absorptiometry (DEXA)

This is a noninvasive diagnostic test obtained in which the patient is exposed to radiation of two distinct intensities (70 and 140 kVp), allowing serial analysis with minimal risk.[3] The precision and accuracy of this technique has been validated in vivo[27–29] and in vitro[30] in several species, including humans. The results obtained correlate well with those obtained using heavy isotope techniques and chemical cadaver analysis.[28] The equipment used (central or peripheral) and the corresponding software allow determination of bone density or quantification of the composition of the different body compartments (e.g. adipose or lean tissue).[3,5] Paediatric and adult software programmes are recommended for pets weighing 5–35 kg and more than 35 kg, respectively. This technique requires appropriate positioning of the patient[13] in dorsal decubitus with the forelimbs against the chest wall (similar to the position used for humans [Fig. 8]), hence the need for deep sedation or anaesthesia.

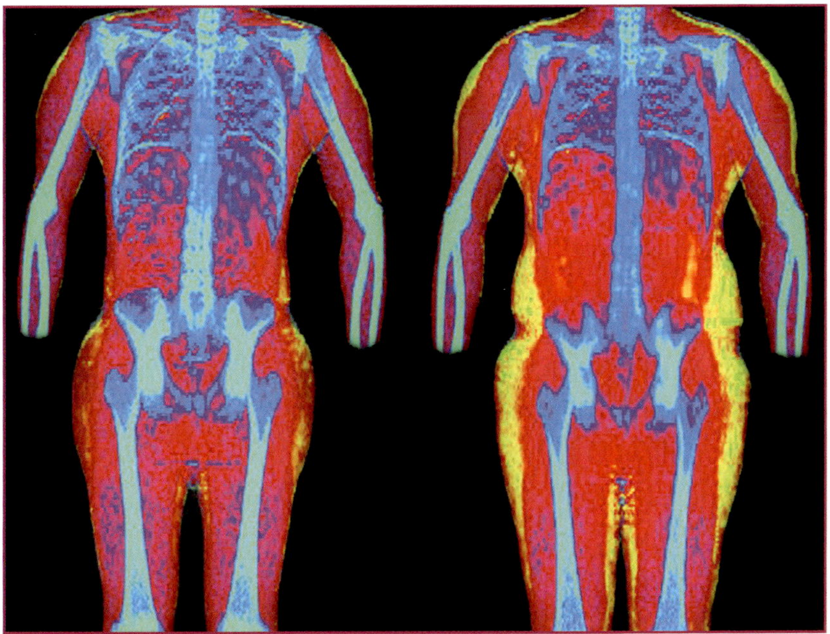

Figure 8. Images obtained by dual-energy X-ray absorptiometry in human medicine.
Yellow, fatty tissue; red/fuchsia, lean tissue; blue, bone.

The mean duration required to obtain images ranges from 20 to 40 minutes, depending on the equipment used. Its use in human medicine is widespread, in contrast to veterinary medicine, where its use is limited owing to its specificity, high cost, and the associated anaesthetic risk.

Computed tomography (CT)

Like DEXA, CT is a method based on diagnostic imaging techniques (Fig. 9). In this case, a three-dimensional image is constructed by computer manipulation of X-rays. Some veterinary clinics have already incorporated CT into their diagnostic equipment. Its use in veterinary studies of body composition is very limited.[9,29,31,32] The results obtained using CT correlate well with those obtained using isotope techniques. The drawbacks are similar to those described for DEXA: expensive equipment and the need to anaesthetise the patient. However, CT allows differentiation between subcutaneous and abdominal fat.

Bioelectrical impedance analysis (BIA)

BIA is a noninvasive method that can be applied in daily clinical practice to estimate body composition.[33] It is based on the Cole–Cole biological impedance model,[34] in which intra- and extracellular water create parallel resistance to the passage of a current. This resistance is directly related to the amount of lean tissue (which consists of 73.2 % water). Because the conductivity of water and muscle is greater than that of fat, the larger the proportion of lean tissue the faster the passage of the current. Conversely, the greater the proportion of adipose tissue in the body, the greater the resistance.

Depending on the species, single or multiple frequency equipment is used. Because the values obtained depend on the degree of hydration and muscle mass, the use of these devices is limited by standardisation, particularly in the case of canids, which comprise numerous breeds. Nonetheless, in both dogs and cats this approach produces results that closely correlate with those obtained using chemical cadaver analysis,[35] DEXA,[4,36] and D_2O.[37–39] Next, a prediction equation is used. The following example is for cats:

$$\text{Body fat (kg)} = -0.05\ \text{Body length (cm)} + 0.7\ \text{Weight (kg)} + 0.007\ \text{Resistance} - 0.60$$

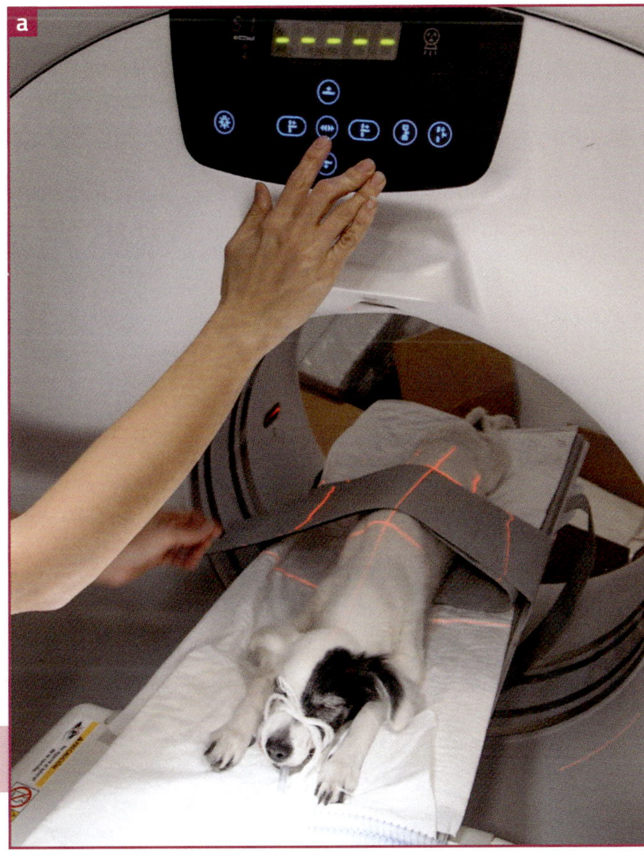

Figure 9. Canine patient during CT study (a and b).

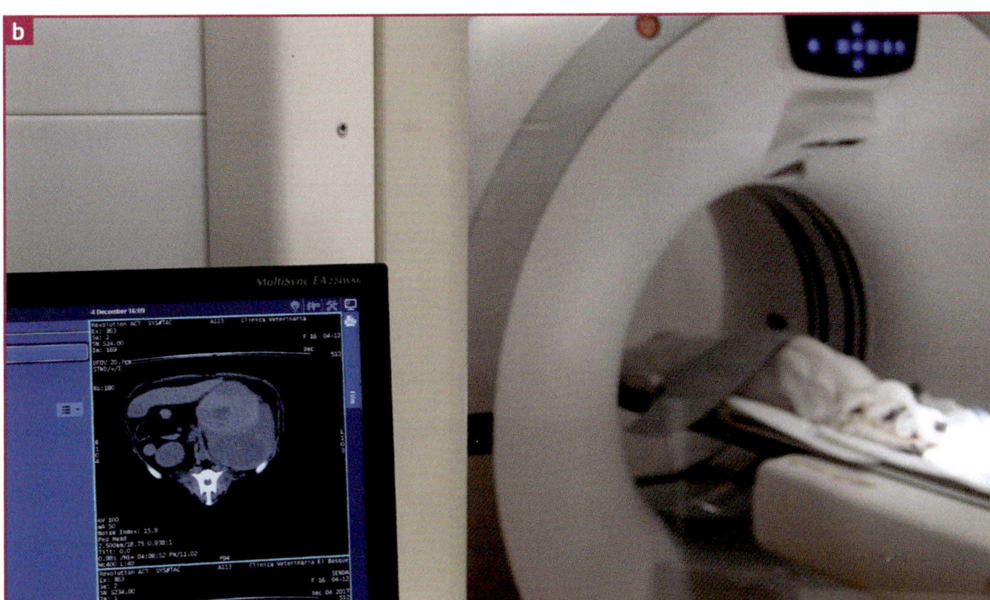

In the case of cats, prediction is somewhat easier owing to the relatively constant size and weight across different breeds.[29]

More studies are needed to validate the different approaches in dogs and cats.

DIAGNOSTIC METHODS IN CLINICAL PRACTICE

Lumbar ultrasound

This is a diagnostic technique used routinely in some clinics, in which ultrasound machines are common. Usually transducers with a frequency of 6–10 MHz are used. Several studies have investigated the correlation between subcutaneous adipose tissue (in different anatomical regions in dogs or cats) and body fat, as determined by chemical composition, DEXA, BIA, morphometric measurements, weight, and BCS.[9,25,29,40,41] Next, using biostatistical analyses, prediction equations are developed. For example, in cats:

$$\text{Body fat (kg)} = 0.3\ \text{Body weight (kg)} + 9.97\ \text{Subcutaneous fat (cm)} - 0.57$$

The distance between the two hyperechoic lines (skin and subcutaneous tissue) provides a measure of subcutaneous fat (hypoechoic line) (Fig. 10). Because different anatomical areas do not show the same correlation the lumbar area, at the level of the third and fifth lumbar vertebrae, is taken as a reference.[25,40] The thickness of subcutaneous fat can vary by more than 50 % (46–83 %) between thin or obese dogs relative to dogs of optimal weight. This technique can detect small variations in subcutaneous fat with high sensitivity.[42] Further research is needed to evaluate different species, breeds, and age groups in order to establish lumbar ultrasound as a reference method.

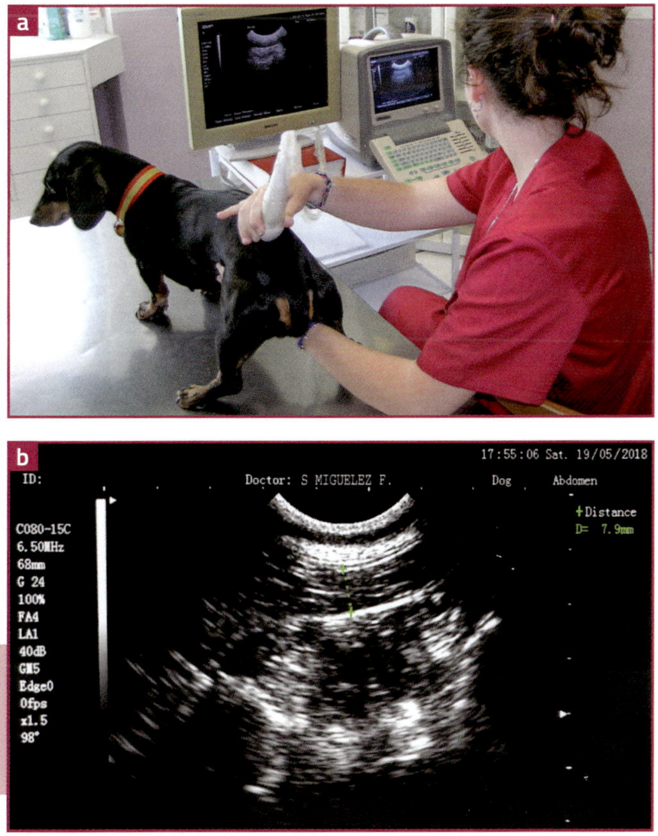

Figure 10. Determination of the thickness of subcutaneous adipose tissue in a patient using lumbar ultrasound (a). Ultrasound image (b).

Morphometric measurements: biometrics

This simple method only requires a measuring tape and a scales. It is based on morphometric studies of the human body. The formulas used can determine body fat content based on current weight and specific body measurements (e.g. pelvic circumference, thoracic circumference, leg length, and height). There are several prediction equations specific to species, age, and sex.[4,16,35,43–47]

The values calculated correlate well with the results obtained by body condition classification, BIA, and DEXA. However, several authors have questioned its validity owing to the fact that repeatability and accuracy are influenced by both patient-related (breed, hair thickness, behavioural profile) and technician-related (experience, selection of measurement points, measuring precision, and tape tension) factors.

Body fat prediction equations

Dogs:

Equation 1	Body fat (%) = $(-0.0034\ HL^2 + 0.0027\ PC^2 - 1.9)/CW$

Equation 2	Body fat (%) = $(-12.937 + 0.696 \times PC)$

Cats:

Equation 3	Body fat (%) = $\{[(TC/0.7067) - HL]/0.9156\} - HL$

Equation 4	Body fat (%) = $66.715 - 0.061 \times (TL^2/CW)$

- HL: right hindlimb length (cm), measured from the calcaneal tuberosity to the middle of the patella (Fig. 11).
- PC: pelvic circumference (cm) at the level of the fifth lumbar vertebra (Fig. 12).
- CW: current weight in kg.
- TC: thoracic circumference at the level of the ninth thoracic vertebra (Fig. 13).
- TL: total length (cm) measured from the tip of the nose to the base of the tail (Fig. 14).

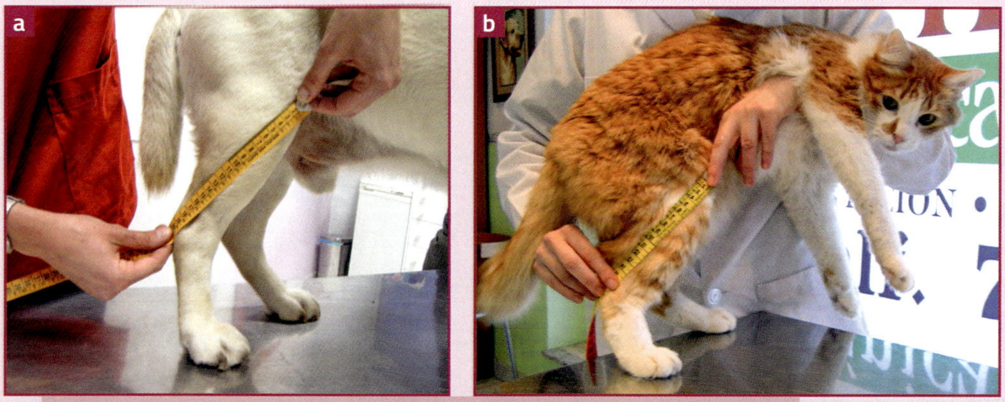

Figure 11. Measurement of the length of the right hindlimb from the calcaneal tuberosity to the middle of the patella in a dog (a) and a cat (b).

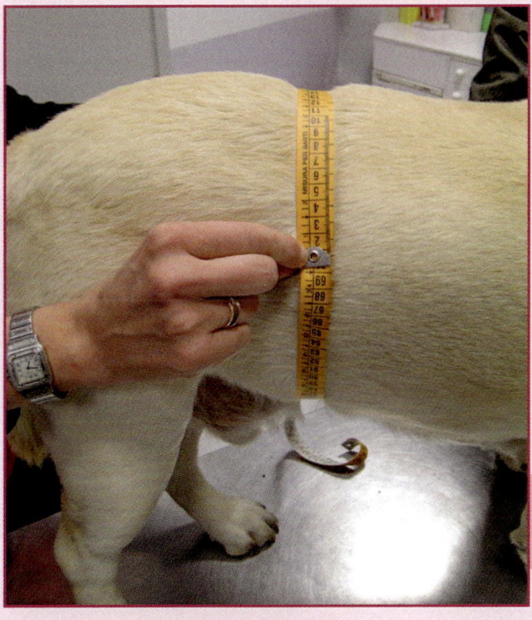

Figure 12. Measurement of the pelvic circumference at the level of the fifth lumbar vertebra in a dog.

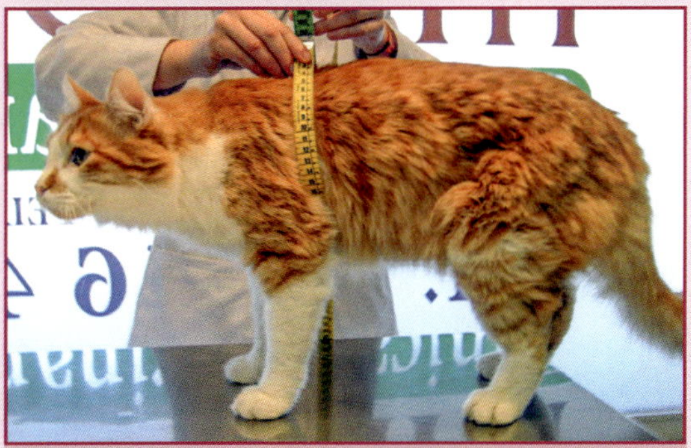

Figure 13. Measurement of the thoracic circumference at the level of the ninth thoracic vertebra in a cat.

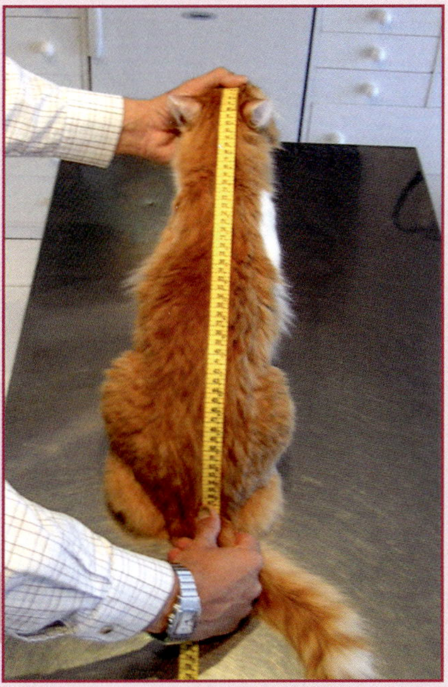

Figure 14. Measurement of the total length from the tip of the nose to the base of the tail in a cat.

Table 2. Parameters evaluated for classification of body condition.

5	9	Classification	Overweight (%)	Ribs (palpation)	Lumbar waist
3/5	5/9	Optimal	0	Light pressure	Evident
4/5	6–7/9	Overweight	+15 (weight increase of 15 %)	Pressure	Moderate
5/5	8–9/9	Obese	>15	Absent	Absent

Body condition score (BCS)

This is the most widespread evaluation system in clinical practice: it is simple, repeatable, reproducible, and easy to learn. It provides a semiquantitative and subjective means of measuring the extent of fat coverage: lateral and dorsal views of the silhouette and palpation of some of the patient's bony prominences (ribs, waist, base of the tail, wing of the ilium, spinous processes of the lumbar vertebrae, chest area) correlate well with the percentage of body fat. A summary is provided in Table 2.

This method has been validated[3,23,28,36,42] using D_2O, BIA, DEXA, and ultrasound techniques, but does not distinguish between canine phenotypes.[4] According to the National Research Council (2006) it is the reference method for determination of the nutritional requirements of dogs and cats.[48] Initially a 5-point scale was used.[49] This has since been updated to a 9-point scale[7,8,12,50,51] (Fig. 15), but may be further modified owing to the increase in the prevalence and severity of morbid obesity (e.g. in cats confined to the home with a BCS of 9/9, body fat percentage can reach 50–55 %[10]). There are other scales based on 3, 4, and 7 points, all of which are similar to those described.

Each point represents a 5 % increase in body fat on the 9-point scale (or a 10 % increase in the case of the 5-point scale). This increase in adipose tissue becomes evident as overweight (overmass), allowing us to establish the patient's target weight and optimal weight. Owing to the scarcity of feline studies, the same values are used as in dogs, despite the differences between the species in the proportions of lean and fatty tissue. Applying equations 5, 6, and 7 (shown below), we obtain the result shown in Table 3.

	Lumbar vertebrae (palpation)	Pectoral area (jugular fossa)	Lateral silhouette	Dorsal silhouette	Abdomen	Base of the tail
	Pressure	Present	Cone-shaped trunk	Infinity symbol	Tucked up	Evident
	Pressure ++	Moderate	Rectangular	Rectangular	Distended	Moderate
	Absent	Absent	Barrel	Barrel	Prominent	Body fat

Less than normal weight

1 Ribs, lumbar vertebrae, pelvis, and other bony prominences are evident. There is no fat and the loss of muscle tissue is notable.

2 The ribs, lumbar vertebrae, pelvic bones, and other bony prominences are easily visible. There is no palpable fat and the loss of muscle mass is minimal.

3 The ribs can be palpated and are easily visible. No fat is detectable by touch. The spinous processes of the lumbar vertebrae are visible and the pelvic bones evident. The abdomen is contracted and the waist visible.

Ideal weight

4 The ribs are easily palpable and have a minimal layer of fat. The waist is dorsally visible. The abdomen is contracted and firm.

5 The ribs can be palpated and lack excess fat. The waist is visible behind the ribs when viewed dorsally. The abdomen is laterally contracted.

Overweight

6 The ribs are palpable and have a light layer of fat. The waist is only visible dorsally, but is not prominent. Some retraction of the abdomen is evident.

7 The ribs can be palpated with difficulty, and there is a thick layer of body fat that is most evident in the lumbar area and at the base of the tail. The waist is absent or barely visible. The abdomen is only slightly retracted.

8 The ribs are only palpable under the thick layer of fat when heavy pressure is applied. There are large fat deposits in the lumbar region and at the base of the tail. The waist is not evident. The abdomen is flaccid and slightly distended.

9 There are very large deposits of fat on the thorax, spinal column, and the base of the tail, and fat on the neck and limbs. The waist is not evident and the abdomen sags.

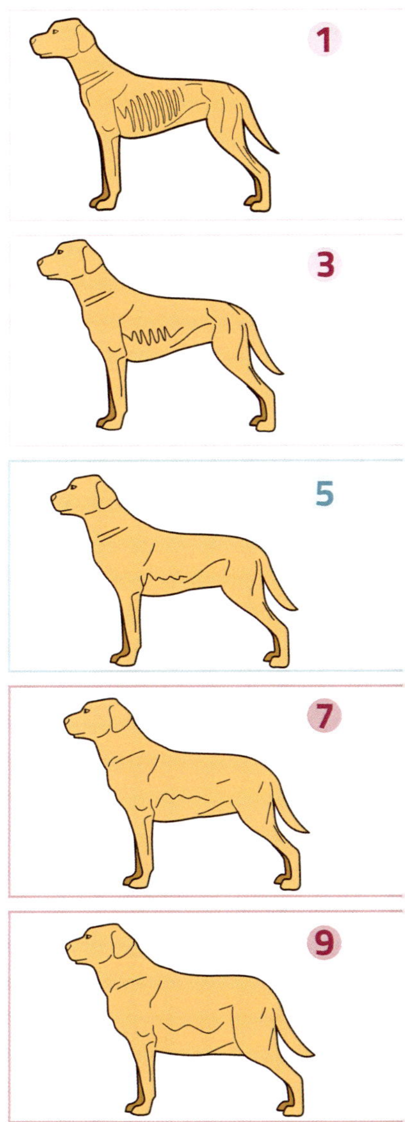

Figure 15. Nine-point scale for the classification of body condition.

Equations for calculating overweight and optimal weight

Equation 5	Overweight (%) = (Current weight × 100/Optimal weight) - 100

Equation 6	Optimal weight (kg) = Current weight × [(100 - % Body fat)/0.8]/100

Equation 7	Optimal $weight_{real/adjusted}$ (kg) = Current weight/(100 - % Overweight) × 100

Table 3. Five- and nine-point scales for BCS, body fat (%), and real (crude) and adjusted overweight (%).

Five-point scale	**3**		**4**		**5**
BF (%)	20		30		≥40
Nine-point scale	**5**	**6**	**7**	**8**	**9**
BF (%)	20	25	30	35	≥40-45
$Overweight_{real}$ (%) *	0	+6.7	+14.3	+23.1	≥33.3
Adjusted overweight (%)	0	+10	+15 (+20)	+25 (+30)	+35 (+40)

* Using Equation 6.

Since it has been determined that the mean lean tissue content is 80 %, each point of the 9-point scale corresponds to an adjusted overweight of 10 percentage points relative to the preceding score, with the exception of scores of 6 and 7, which reflect increases of 5 points relative to the preceding score (Equation 7). To facilitate calculations, increments of 10 % are used (parentheses in Table 3).

Biochemical markers

This in vitro method allows quantification of body fat based on classification of body condition, which is determined based on weight and several different blood parameters.[52,53] Regression analysis was used to select, from a variety of analyses regularly performed in veterinary clinics, the parameters necessary for classification of dogs using a 5-point scale: urea, sodium, and chlorine levels. The corresponding prediction formula is shown below (Equation 8):

Equation 8	BCS = 3.64120 + (0.18614 × Body weight in kg) - (0.05289 × Urea in mg/dl) + (0.08935 × Sodium in mmol/l) - (0.14088 × Chlorine in mmol/l)

Other prediction equations use other parameters that are less common/standardised in clinical practice (e.g. C-reactive protein and the hormone TSH).

Although good results have been obtained, more studies are required in both species and in other breeds to validate the systematic use of these parameters.

Example

Sarastro is an 8-year-old, castrated mixed-breed dog with a current weight of 29 kg. After performing biometrics (HL = 21 cm; PC = 69.5 cm) a BCS of 8/9 is calculated (Fig. 16). What is the recommended/optimal weight and percentage body fat?

Equation 1	Body fat (%) = (0.0034 HL^2 + 0.0027 PC^2 - 1.9)/CW Body fat (%) = [(-0.0034 × 21^2) + (0.0027 × 69.5^2) - 1.9)]/29 × 100	35.44 %	Mean: 34.6 %
Equation 2	Body fat (%) = (-12.937 + 0.696 × PC) Body fat (%) = (-12.937 + 0.696 × 69.5)	33.25 %	
BCS	7/9	35 %	
Equation 5	Overweight (%) = (Current weight × 100/Optimal weight) - 100 Overweight (%) = (29 × 100/23.6) – 100	23.1 %	Mean: 23.4 kg
Equation 6	Optimal weight (kg) = Current weight × [(100 - % Body fat)/0.8]/100 Optimal weight (kg) = 29 × [(100 - 34.6)/0.8]/100	23.7 kg	
Equation 7	Optimal weight$_{real}$ (kg) = Current weight/(100 - % Overweight) × 100 Optimal weight$_{real}$ = 29/(100 - 23.1) × 100	23.6 kg	
Equation 7	Adjusted optimal weight (kg) = Current weight/(100 - % Overweight) × 100 Adjusted optimal weight= 29/(100 - 25) × 100	23.2 kg	

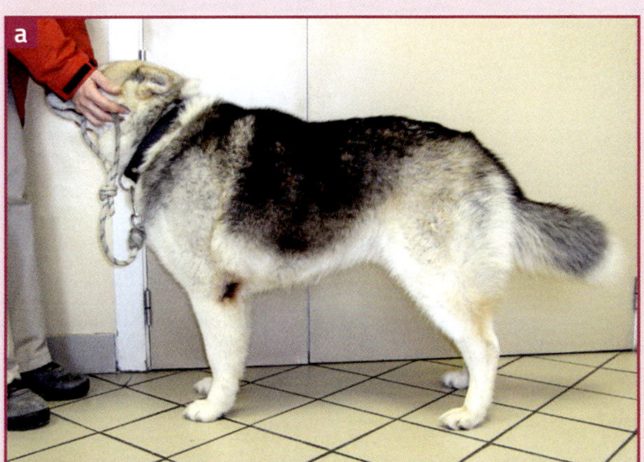

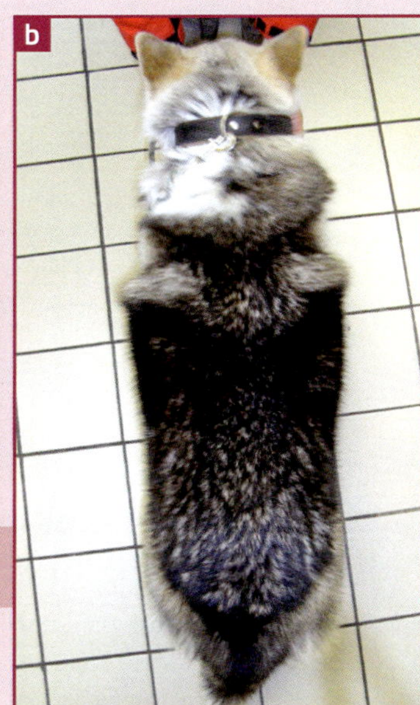

Figure 16. Patient during body condition assessment (a). Appearance from dorsoventral view (b).

4 Communication with owners

INTRODUCTION

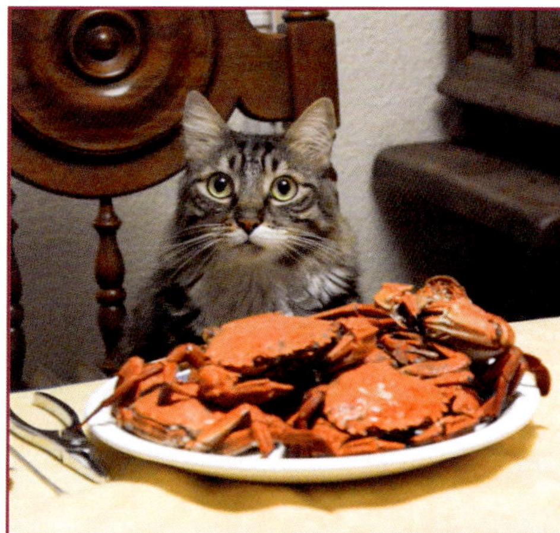

Figure 1. The humanisation of pets results in a loss of objectivity as to their real needs.

The growing tendency to humanise pets puts veterinary practitioners in a difficult situation when explaining to an owner that their "little friend" is obese and therefore ill (Fig. 1). The owner can view their pet's condition from two different perspectives: anthropocentrism (i.e. "it's a dog/cat, nothing more") or biocentrism (i.e. "all living beings have the same rights"). This is until they are presented with the costs of diagnosis and treatment. Indeed, 10 % of owners believe that treatments are prescribed for economic reasons.[1] In these situations, the natural tendency of the clinician is to minimise the seriousness of the animal's condition, thereby contravening our Hippocratic oath or deontological code. This is a source of frustration and work-related anxiety for some veterinary surgeons, who would prefer to avoid such uncomfortable situations. However, it is our professional responsibility to deal with obesity as we would any other disease.

On the other hand, it seems contradictory to create laws to protect animal welfare[2] while ignoring overweight, which, in any species, constitutes a form of abuse.

Whether the owner likes it or not, obesity is a disease that diminishes the pet's life expectancy and quality of life.[3]

INTERACTION WITH THE OWNER

We are faced with a complex, sensitive, and multi-faceted issue that requires the participation of the entire clinical team (veterinary assistants and specialists in different areas of veterinary medicine). Before proposing a weight-loss programme we must be sure that we have the conviction, trust, complicity, and participation of the pet owner. The following are two key concepts:

- Conviction: the ability to comprehend the seriousness of the disease and our treatment recommendations.
- Trust: the ability to adhere to the recommended treatment programme (Fig. 2).

This will determine the level of commitment to and the success of the weight-loss programme.

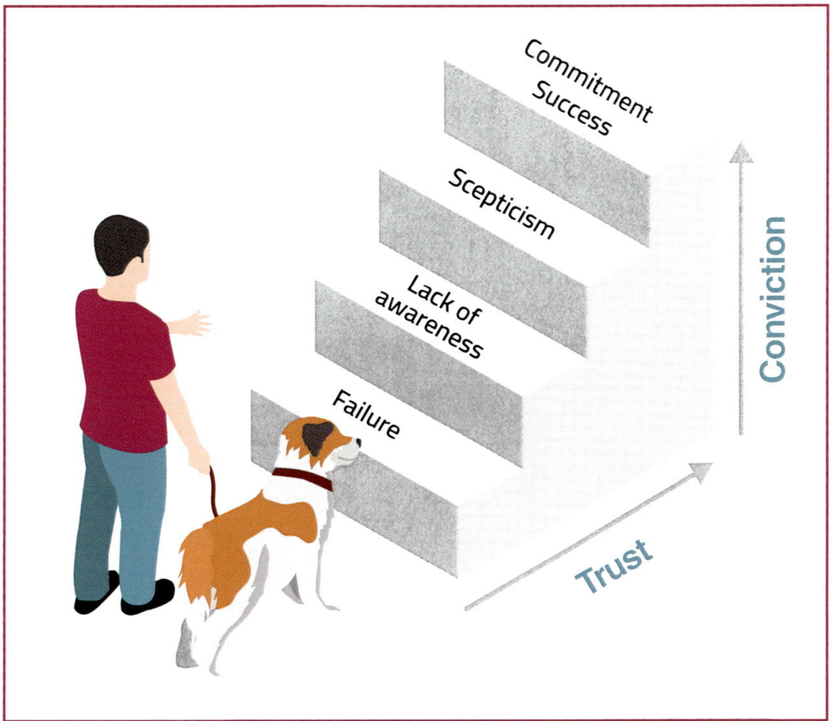

Figure 2. Motivational keys for successful application of a weight-loss programme.

Two types of relationship between the medical professional and the patient (in our case, the pet owner) are described: a relationship based on deference to the recommendations of the doctor or veterinary surgeon, and a relationship whereby the two parties interact in order to reach an agreement. These are two opposing relationships; obedience versus participation (Fig. 3). The World Health Organization recognises the benefit of the second option.[4] Identifying obstacles and working through them with the owner to develop an action plan is highly beneficial. We must not forget that the owner needs to understand the health-disease binomial (including the prognosis) and the different treatment options, since they themselves play an active role in each stage of their pet's life.

A 2003 study reported that, in theory, 59 % of owners comply with the dietary recommendations proposed by their clinical team. The reality, however, is quite different: only 21 % adhere to these recommendations. Moreover, 55 % of "compliant owners" offer additional food (home-cooked food,

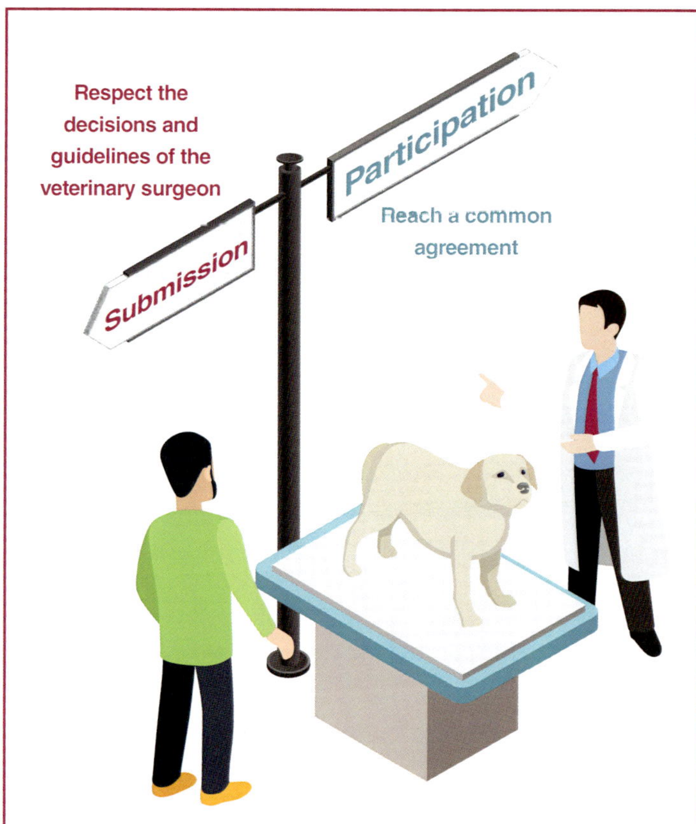
Respect the decisions and guidelines of the veterinary surgeon
Participation
Reach a common agreement
Submission

Figure 3. Relationships that can be established between the owner and the veterinary surgeon.

rewards, etc.) to their pets.[1] An owner can comply with our recommendations regarding the strict application of a specific diet for their obese pet, but will stop collaborating if they perceive that their dog or cat does not like the food. The owner's perception of a given diet is dependent on their personal preferences, which they extrapolate to their pet, and on the manner in which their pet has been trained (altered feeding behaviour can lead to a capricious appetite). Here we must attempt to balance the perception of the disease, the interests of the patient, and the responsibility of the owner. Therefore, we should not attempt to force the owner to comply; this is a more appropriate approach in the context of legally required procedures (e.g. when chipping the pet or administering a rabies vaccine), but not for the case at hand. Nor should we provide the client with multiple options and leave the decision to them.

Models

Psychologists have proposed several systems to explain how changes in our behaviours can lead to improvement. For example:

- The transtheoretical model of change of Prochaska and Diclemente (1982)[5] (Fig. 4).
- The E4 model of Keller and Carroll (1994).[6]
- Four Habits, by Frankel and Stein (1996).[7]
- The ADOBE model, by Carroll and Goldstein (2003).[8]

Their use in veterinary medicine can help improve the quality of the consultation, particularly by facilitating collaboration and resolving conflict (Fig. 5) between the owner and veterinary practitioner (or patient and doctor), which arises in 30 % of cases.[9]

In general, all these models propose a series of steps necessary to achieve the complicity of the owner, although each requires some degree of flexibility on the part of the clinician.

Investigate the cause and address the problem

As a first point of contact, we should evaluate the type of patient and attempt to gain the trust of the owner. Our attitude towards the owner should make them feel unique. It is essential to listen carefully to the information they provide about the pet, since it is the owner who spends most of their day with the pet. When performing the anamnesis, we should avoid a strict or pre-defined set of questions and try to use a broader questioning approach. While this may take longer than usual, the consultation will be well performed, and the

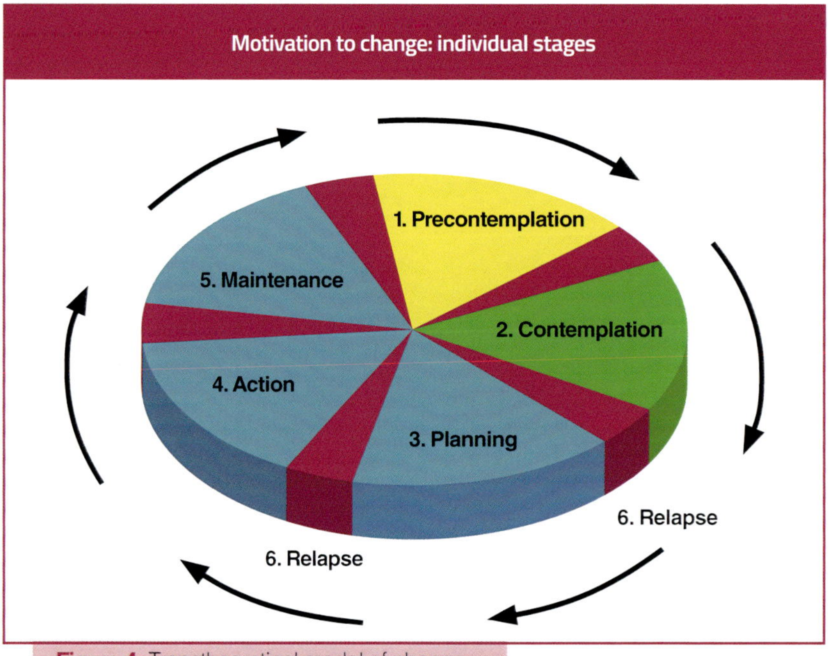

Figure 4. Transtheoretical model of change (Prochaska and Diclemente, 1982).

owner will feel safe and well received and will pay more attention to our explanations. The owner may tell us that their dog does not eat much, which is probably not true. Nonetheless, we should persevere, bearing in mind that the owner is likely unaware of their pet's condition. We may hear explanations such as: "it's winter and he has more hair", "she's not obese, it's pure muscle", "he's a Labrador", "he's castrated", "she has that pretty little face and never stops pleading for food when we're eating" or "it's only a few kilos, but he's so happy... "

It is very important that we control our emotions at this point; we should not repeat ourselves or change our tone, and if we feel that we will lose control it is better to leave the office for a few minutes, take a breath, and return. Recognising body language during the consultation can help. Signs of defence include crossed arms, hugging of the pet, increasing the distance from the veterinary professional or positioning oneself on the other side of the examination table, speaking louder and enunciating certain words, body tension, and frowning.[10,11]

When faced with a continuous lack of cooperation on the part of the owner, indicating that they are not yet ready for change, it is preferable to

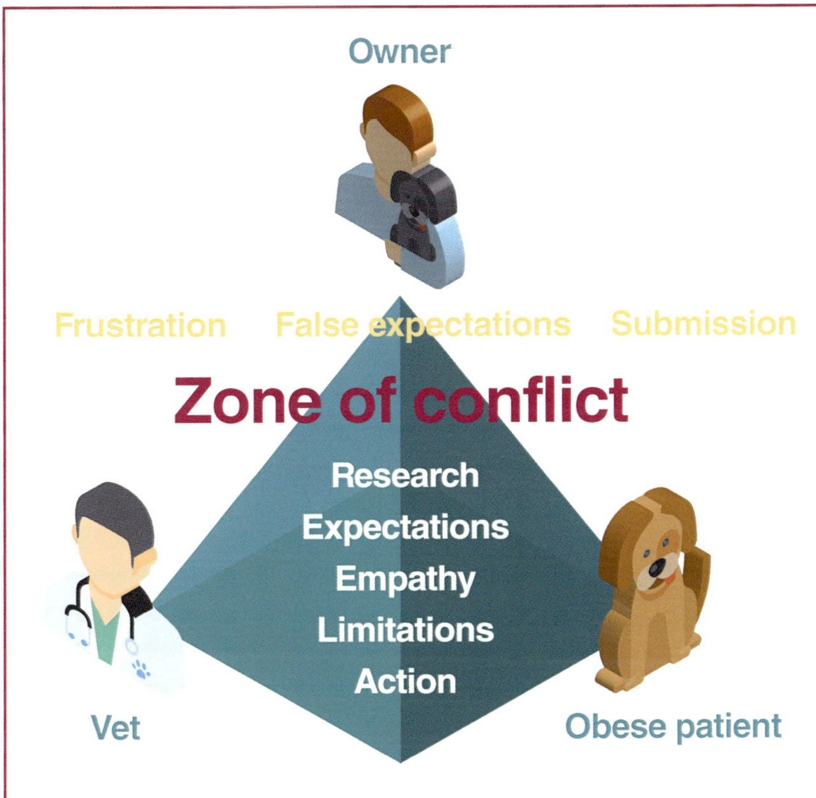

Figure 5. Zone of conflict in the owner-vet relationship.

schedule an appointment for 30 to 60 days later, when the issue can be re-addressed. Success in obesity programmes depends on patient care and follow-up.

The issue can be brought up initially in the context of a regular checkup. For example, if while completing the patient's clinical history the veterinary surgeon or assistant (or trainee student) says "temperature, mucous membranes, pulse..., weight = x kg, body score = 8/9, obese..." it is very likely that the owner will ask us what this means. We could then begin the therapeutic approach, informing the owner that their pet is overweight by x kg, but could lose this weight within a certain number of months. It is not necessary to say "he's a little overweight", "we should think about putting him on a diet", or "we'll discuss it another day". We must be proactive in addressing the issue with the owner.

Understand the owner's expectations

We are at a stage at which the owner has already acknowledged the disease. The owner has reconsidered, and starts asking us questions. Now is when we must provide information about obesity and determine what sort of outcome the owner expects. We must consider the owner's opinions. From this point, the veterinary team and the owner decide upon the course of action to be taken.

As we provide more information and offer more treatment alternatives, the pet owner will become more involved in the project, and the likelihood of misunderstandings will decrease. This is how conviction is reaffirmed.

Show empathy

Empathy is required in order to better understand the owner. We have to determine their perspective of their pet's condition. It helps if we ourselves are also dog or cat owners. It should be borne in mind that we may encounter owners with erroneous beliefs resulting from information they find online (about 17 %) or acquire from their peers (especially other dog owners that they meet in the park). According to a recent Canadian study, only 7 % of veterinary surgeons show empathy towards their clients.[12]

What if the owner is obese? What if we are obese? There are two situations that can arise. In the first case, the appropriate approach is to simply focus exclusively on the pet's condition, informing the owner about the benefits of a healthy weight. Do not respond to any comments by the owner comparing the pet's weight to their own ("he's chubby like me"); continue focusing on the health and well-being of the patient, and not on the number of kilos of overweight (this will be addressed once the owner understands the expected outcome). In the second case, we can look for empathy by mentioning that, like the patient, we are addressing our own overweight in order to improve our life expectancy and quality of life, and then redirect the conversation to focus on the patient's illness. Statements such as "my weight or body condition are unrelated to my professional activity" should be avoided.

Understand the limitations

In some cases, treatment will require owners to carry out certain actions that they will find difficult. For example, the time a dog spends exercising may be conditioned by the age of the owner (elderly owners) or by physical limitations (orthopaedic disease); it may be difficult to modify certain habits (offering extra food outside of meal times); or owners may have economic difficulties. In each and every case, we must attempt to find a solution, such as:

proposing that they find a dog walker; modifying the way they reward their pet; or providing flexible payment options for the animal's treatment. Identifying and recognising the limitations of our recommendations will improve our relationship with the owner, as well as the patient's quality of care.[13]

Final decisions and action

This is a critical phase because it requires discipline on the part of the owner and strict follow-up on the part of the veterinary surgeon. We begin by clearly planning the guidelines to be followed, taking expectations into account, and proceed by instituting treatment and maintaining it over time (generally a weight-loss programme for patients with a BCS of 7/9 will last a minimum of 6 months) until the target weight is reached. At some point during the planning, action, and maintenance steps the owner may reject the approach taken, taking us back to square one.

TYPES OF PET OWNERS

In our daily practice, we will likely encounter three different types of owners, with two distinct backgrounds. These profiles should be considered when deciding how to present information to the owner. Owners can perceive their pet's obesity in three different ways:

- They are aware of the seriousness of the situation: this type of owner is in the minority, accounting for about 2 % of cases.
- They only recognise the secondary pathologies associated with their pet's obesity: these cases are relatively easy to work with. For example: a dog with orthopaedic problems and a BCS of 8/9 who finds it difficult to walk due to the presence of masses on the medial aspect of the right hindlimb and the right shoulder area (Figs. 6 and 7), or a cat with type 2 diabetes and a BCS of 8/9 (Fig. 8).
- They refuse to accept that their pet is ill: these account for 75–80 % of clients. About 53 % agree with the 7/9 score that the veterinary surgeon assigns their dog, although 61 % fail to recognise that their dog's weight is abnormal[14–17] (e.g. *Tosca* "is big boned, like her father" according to the owner of the dog in Fig. 9). In the case of cats, 51 % of owners fail to recognise that their pet is ill.[18,19] Data indicate that 20–40 % of pets living in developed countries are overweight/obese. These figures resemble those reported for paediatric populations: 63 % of parents estimate that their child's body mass index is lower than it actually is.[20,21]

In terms of background, owners fall into two categories:

- Those with an understanding of health.
- Those with little respect for the clinical environment.

Some owners have insufficient capacity to acquire, process, and understand basic health information that allows them to make appropriate decisions for their pets. It is estimated that 25–60 % of adults, particularly those over 60 years of age, have inadequate training in this area.[22] How can we recognise them? These are usually the owners who ask us to repeat the treatment several times and do not take notes or request any written information. They trust their memory. Given this situation, it may be advisable to provide written recommendations.

Given the potential profiles of our clients and the recommended strategies for interacting with them, how should we explain obesity? Should we use

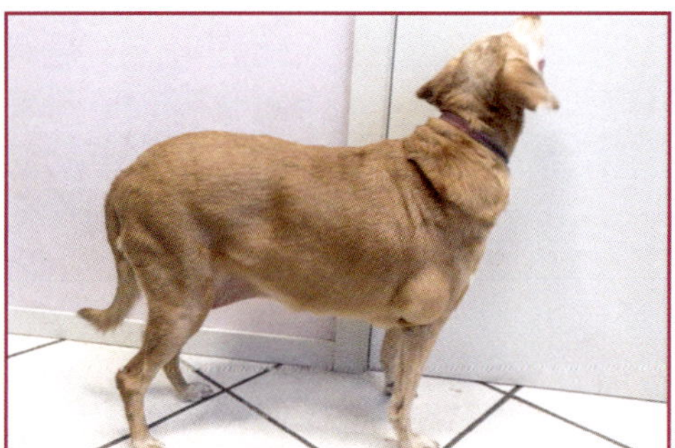

Figure 6. Patient with a BCS of 8/9. A fatty nodule is evident on the right shoulder.

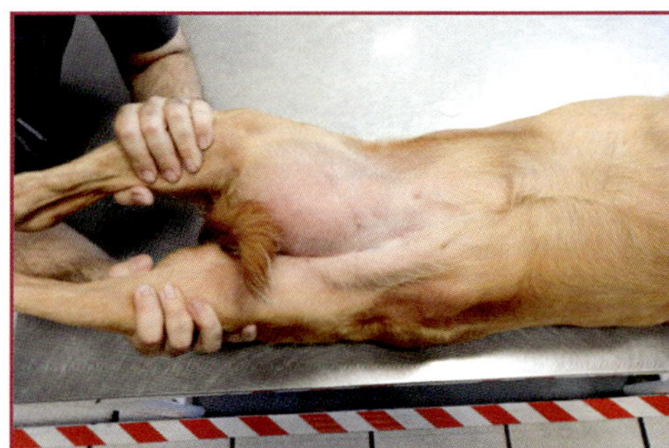

Figure 7. Patient from previous figure. There is an evident accumulation of fat in the right thigh.

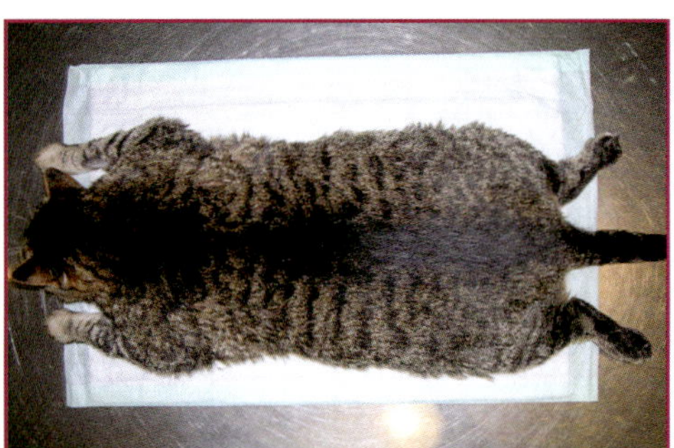

Figure 8. Cat (BCS 8/9) with type 2 diabetes.

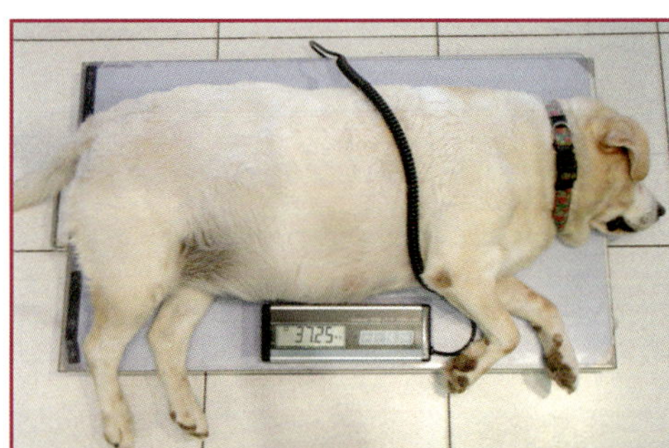

Figure 9. Dog with obvious overweight.

medical terminology or attempt to make medical concepts more easily understandable? In our opinion, it is better to avoid excessive use of technical terminology, and instead to use simpler language to describe the condition. Information should be provided in small blocks, demonstrating (not describing) how the treatment should be applied, leaving appropriate intervals to allow the information to sink in and to monitor the owner's attitude. This will give us an idea of their capacity to adhere to the recommendations. For example, take the case of a cat who should consume 60 g of a specific food daily. In in the clinic in front of the owner, we can weigh out the required amount on a scales and place it in a transparent container, indicating the appropriate level with a marker.

How should the veterinary surgeon deal with the pet owner?

For our part, there are certain points that should be taken into account when dealing with pet owners:

- We must be honest. The treatments in question are long-lasting and require great effort from those in the pet's environment.
- Realistic: we must describe the facts as they are. We must not suggest that we can perform miracles. Results will only be achieved if all those in the pet's environment are focused on a successful outcome.
- Bear in mind that each patient is unique, and requires an individualised treatment for weight loss.
- We should offer the owner a smile and a positive attitude.
- We must be patient and offer our work time without interruption.
- Never make the owner feel guilty.
- Do not use offensive words (e.g. fat, chubby) or general expressions (e.g. "I've seen fatter" or "many pets need to lose weight").
- We must emphasise the benefits of a healthy weight and conformation and prioritise the health and well-being of the pet.
- All information should be provided in the consultation room. Never treat an overweight patient in the waiting room (the owner may feel uncomfortable in the presence of other owners) or discuss the patient when saying goodbye at the clinic door (e.g. a veterinary surgeon remarking "let's talk about this little fat fellow next week"). These actions indicate a lack of seriousness towards the patient's condition.
- The patient should always be seen by the veterinary surgeon responsible for nutrition, leaving the assistants to perform initial evaluations in follow-up visits and to coordinate subsequent appointments.

5 Nutrients in weight-loss programmes

The digestion products of the three main nutrients have effects, both direct and indirect (via endocrine regulation), on the control of ingestion and energy metabolism. As such, the role of macronutrients in the treatment of overweight/obese patients is one of the most controversial areas of nutrition, particularly in human medicine, owing to the multitude of diets with varying macronutrient content and distribution. Consider, for example, the Dukan, Atkins, or Montignac diets.

The basis of any weight-loss programme is to reduce energy intake while ensuring that the remaining nutrients meet the energy requirements of the species. Since the energy is conserved, the metabolisable energy corresponding to a unit of lost weight is equivalent to the energy deficit necessary to lose weight. Accordingly, the basis of any weight-loss programme is a reduction in the ingestion of the most energetic nutrients, ensuring that the remaining nutrients cover the needs of the species in question. This principle is valid for both prescription foods and for homemade diets recommended by veterinary surgeons. For this reason, commercial foods formulated to fulfil the maintenance requirements of healthy animals should be avoided as they could result in deficiencies and will not satiate the patient, potentially frustrating the owner.

Next we will discuss in more detail some of the nutrients implicated in weight-loss programmes.

ENERGY

As mentioned above, the first step in combatting uncontrolled ingestion of food is to reduce caloric intake while maintaining the volume of the digestive system. This can be achieved by diluting the ration (altering the moisture and fibre content of the product) or by reducing energy (primarily by targeting fat content).

Stomach capacity in dogs and cats

The stomach volume of a dog or cat is approximately 5–10 ml/kg live weight, although capacities of 45–90 ml/kg after feeding are described.[1,2] Analysis of these figures shows that the capacity of the stomach ranges from 1 % to 9 % of the animal's weight (Fig. 1). Commercial foods are formulated using the highest values (4–9 % of body weight) in the case of wet formulations (cans) and lower values (1–2 % of body weight) in the case of dry feed (kibble): the volume (weight) is inversely correlated to the amount of dry matter in the food.

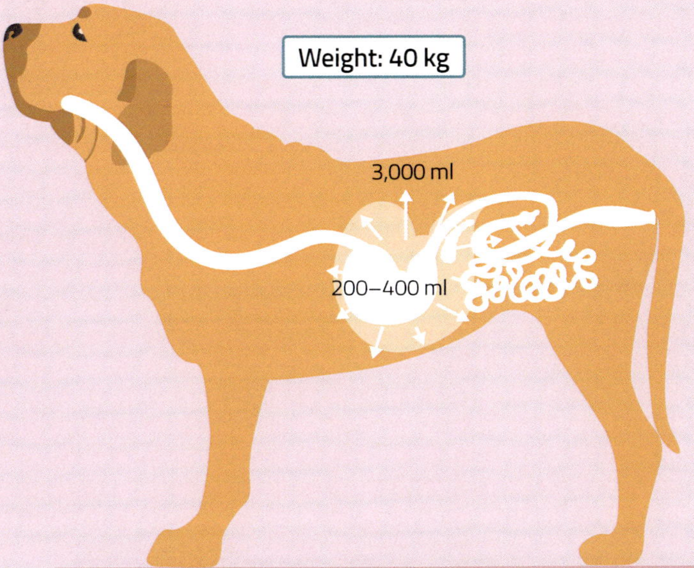

Figure 1. Fluctuation of a dog's stomach capacity.

Most commercial foods have an energy content ranging from 900 to 3,900 kcal of metabolisable energy per kg of food (≈4,000 kcal ME/kg DM). This value must be taken into account when adjusting the volume of the ration to the previously calculated values. Nutrient content is adjusted to correspond to this energy content (i.e. to achieve a balanced kilocalorie intake).

Example

If we offer a 15-kg dog dry feed (9 % moisture content) containing 3,700 kcal ME/kg of feed, the daily complete and balanced ration will be approximately 270 g, or 1.8 % of body weight.

When treating an obese patient, it is important to attempt to maintain volume while reducing the energy density and to increase the amounts of other nutrients in the ration. To this end, prescription or dietetic foods with a specific objective are used:[3,4] in this case, foods indicated for "reduction of excess weight, obesity, or overweight" (or similar). All such products must indicate the corresponding energetic content and include a warning indicating that consultation with a veterinary surgeon is recommended before use, except in cases of prescription foods and those indicated for use for specific nutritional purposes. Most commercially available products have an energy concentration of 3,000 kcal ME/kg of food (≤3,400 kcal ME/kg DM).

Exceptions include some dietetic foods for the treatment of feline diabetes and associated obesity, the metabolisable energy content of which is close to 3,800 kcal ME/kg (4,000 kcal ME/kg DM). The legislation covering these foods is identical to that described above.

These products should not be confused with foods that claim to be "low-calorie", "light", or "reduced calories". Several private organisations propose a code of good practice for the production of animal food, as well as labelling guidelines (e.g. the Fédération Européenne de l'Industrie des Aliments pour Animaux Familiers – FEDIAF – in Europe[5] and the Association of American Feed Control Officials – AAFCO – in the United States[6]).

According to these organisations, this type of food should have a reduction in energy content of at least 15 %, or should indicate the percentage reduction (per unit dry matter) relative to another standard food of similar nutritional characteristics. Although the energy density of these products may be close to that of prescription diets, they are not recommended for the treatment of obese patients. Certification by these organisations can be viewed as a form of quality assurance.

Generally, caloric content is decreased by reducing lipid content. This does not mean that "low-fat" foods are exclusively for the treatment of obese patients, as discussed further below.

The use of semi-moist food (14–60 % moisture content) or wet food (moisture content >60 %) is a useful strategy. As the proportion of water in the food increases, the nutrient content is diluted and there is an added physiological effect on the receptors of the wall of the digestive system. However, the use of these foods is restricted to cats and small dog breeds owing to their composition (simple carbohydrates such as fructose and sorbitol act as humectants), the space required for storage, and the price per unit of dry matter.

There are no specific recommendations as regards the energy content of any of the aforementioned products.

FAT AND FAT-SOLUBLE NUTRIENTS

Fat is the main nutrient that is restricted in foods intended for obese patients. The reasons are several (Fig. 2).

Figure 2. Triglyceride, composed of one molecule of glycerol and three chains of saturated fatty acids (molekuul_be, Shutterstock.com).

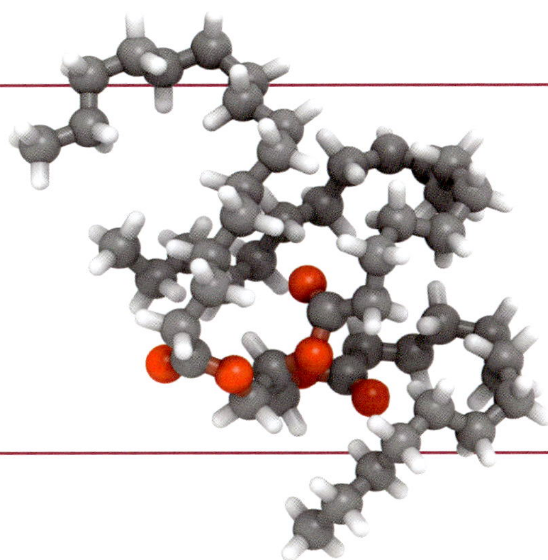

Nutritional characteristics of fat that necessitate its restriction in weight-control programmes:

- Provides almost 2.5 times more energy than protein and hydrates.
- High digestibility (>90 %).
- High utilisation efficiency (0.86–0.95).
- Low thermogenic effect.

However, we must remember that fats are necessary components of all diets, given their important structural (e.g. myelin), metabolic (essential fatty acids), and functional (e.g. transport of fat-soluble vitamins and regulation of prostaglandins and eicosanoids) roles. Furthermore, they directly affect the palatability and texture of the food, and therefore influence voluntary ingestion.

Some authors have reported greater weight loss in dogs fed on low-fat versus high-fat diets,[7] as well as maintenance of weight and body fat despite reduced caloric intake in animals fed on fat-rich diets.[8] However, research in humans offers a contradictory perspective: results obtained after a minimum of 12 months and a maximum of 24 months of treatment revealed no statistically significant differences between high- and low-fat diets,[9] with the exception of ultra-low-fat diets.[10] Regardless of the levels of the predominant macronutrient in a given diet, weight will always be lost when the number of calories consumed is reduced:[8] high-fat diets with an approximate reduction in calories of 35 % result in weight loss similar to that observed with low-fat diets, while maintaining good cardiovascular health. Therefore, low-fat food is not synonymous with low-calorie food.

Analysis of prescription diets designed for the treatment of obese patients reveals that they provide 30–38 g of fat/1,000 kcal ME, with the exception of some products for obese and diabetic cats that contain 45–50 g fat/1,000 kcal ME. Comparison of these products with those intended to fulfil the maintenance requirements of healthy adult animals shows that, in many cases, there is little difference in fat content per unit of energy.

According to the recommendations of FEDIAF and AAFCO, commercially available "low-fat" foods should contain 20–30 g of fat/1,000 kcal ME. They can also be used for patients with other diseases (e.g. pancreatitis) or for enteral feeding.

There are no recommendations regarding the appropriate level of fat when formulating a prescription diet. The National Research Council (NRC, 2006)[11] recommends 13.8 and 22.5 g of fat/1,000 kcal ME for dogs and cats, respectively. These values are lower than those found in prescription foods and those intended for adults.

Polyunsaturated fatty acids

As discussed in Chapter 2, proinflammatory cytokines (e.g. interleukins, tumour necrosis factor α) are released in obese patients. The lipid content of the ration, particularly that of eicosapentaenoic (EPA), docosapentaenoic (DPA), and docosahexaenoic (DHA) omega-3 fatty acids, plays an important role in the control of this process. Via their biological mediators (resolvins E and D and protectins) they regulate the production of certain interleukins and associated factors, blocking the migration of leukocytes to the inflammatory focus,[12] modifying the structure of the membrane and making it less proinflammatory (e.g. replacing arachidonic acid – AA – with α-linolenic acid – ALA –), or competitively inhibiting lipoxygenases and cyclooxygenases.[11] On the other hand, studies in rodents have shown that high dietary levels (up to 21 g of omega-3/1,000 kcal ME) increase adiponectin levels, suggesting that this constitutes a potential strategy for the treatment of obesity.

Dogs and cats lack the ability to elongate and desaturate fatty acids to form the polyunsaturated omega-3 fatty acids ALA, EPA, and DHA. For this reason, these fatty acids are included in diets for obese patients, although their effect in veterinary medicine remains unclear. While there is little information available regarding their benefits in these diets, the NRC[11] recommends 0.11 g and 0.025 g of EPA + DHA/1,000 kcal ME for dogs and cats, respectively. Most commercial maintenance or prescription diets follow the recommendations of the NRC, respecting the limits of toxicity: fatty acid levels can be 4–10 times the recommended value. In certain prescription foods, reporting of the EPA and DHA content is mandatory.[4] In our case, the minimum content should be 0.4 g EPA + DHA/1,000 kcal ME (Fig. 3).

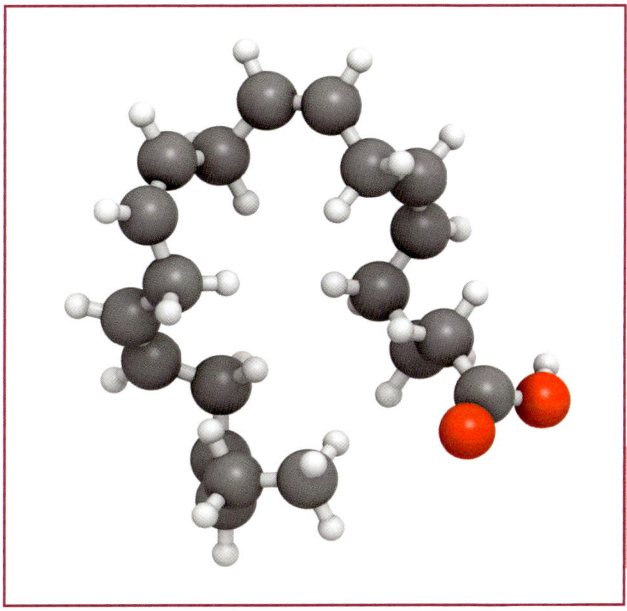

Figure 3. Molecule of eicosapentaenoic (EPA) omega-3 fatty acid (molekuul_be, Shutterstock.com).

Vitamin E and selenium

These two nutrients act synergistically against cellular oxidation. Vitamin E (α-tocopherol is the most active isomer) does so in the cell membrane, targeting polyunsaturated fatty acids, while selenium is found in glutathione-peroxidase and acts within the cytoplasm. Its presence in diets for obese pets is intimately linked to the nature of the chronic process (in which oxidative damage occurs),[13] possible fatty degeneration of the liver,[14,15,16] and the increased levels of some polyunsaturated fatty acids (PUFAs) in prescription foods (e.g. in salmon- or tuna-based products or those containing fish oils).[17,18] Vitamin E is a safe and widely used vitamin, the presence of which must be declared on the product label.[4]

The recommended amount of vitamin E varies depending on the ingestion of PUFAs and the PUFA content of the ration. With higher levels of PUFA ingestion, a greater amount of vitamin E will be required to stabilise the membranes and act as an antioxidant: it is recommended to maintain a ratio of 0.6–1.2 mg per gram of fatty acid per kg of food.

Owing to the many different commercially available brands for the management of overweight pets, recommended amounts can vary widely (by up to 15 or 20 fold), even in maintenance formulas.

In the case of selenium, some authors recommend a minimum of a 45 % increase with respect to values recommended by the NRC for prescription diets (i.e. 0.125 mg/1,000 kcal ME). These figures remain well below the upper safety limit (0.5 mg/1,000 kcal ME).[11]

FIBRE

The addition of fibre is the method traditionally used to dilute the energy content of a product.[19] Fibre serves another function in the diets of obese patients by controlling the voluntary ingestion of food and modifying the digestibility and absorption in the digestive system of certain nutrients.[20–23]

Fibre delays gastric emptying, decreases the passage of chyme, and increases intestinal transit time. In general, it increases total gastrointestinal transit time (thus increasing the interval between meals). In addition, by inducing gastric distension it triggers the release of hormones that also modulate appetite. Its effects will depend on the predominant type of fibre (fermentable or nonfermentable) and its levels in the diet.[24]

Defining exactly how fibre influences satiety is challenging, since satiety is a subjective concept and is difficult to assess in pets, especially when their natural eating behaviour has been altered. Research in this field has produced varying results.[25–30]

The incorporation of fibre into the ration reduces energy digestibility by almost 10 %. The underlying mechanisms involve the formation of insoluble complexes or the inhibition of enzymes responsible for metabolism.[21,22,30–33] It is important to consider the role of fibre in the metabolism of carbohydrates and cholesterol: its presence helps to control blood glucose levels and maintain cardiovascular health.[31,33,34]

Of the different nutrients implicated in weight-loss programmes for companion animals, fibre is one of the first to be considered when prescribing food to the patient.

Fibre is directly responsible for flatulence and the frequency, volume, and consistency of the faeces, and therefore results in modification of the animal's defecation habits, a phenomenon to which owners continually attest. These effects will be determined by the type of fibre selected: fermentable fibre produces softer stools and an increase in the frequency of defecation as compared with insoluble fibre.[22] For these reasons, most commercial fibre-rich foods for obese patients predominantly contain insoluble fibre. It is important to remember to inform the owner of the pros and cons of a specific dietary programme.

The NRC has no established recommendations regarding fibre content. Studies indicate that the amount of crude fibre in food products formulated to prevent weight gain or promote weight loss in dogs and cats varies from 35 to 60 g of fibre/1,000 kcal ME, with a proportion of 20 % fermentable fibre.

It is mandatory to indicate the raw fibre content of the product on the label.[3] However, this only reflects the amount of insoluble fibre, and therefore underestimates the actual fibre content. It would be more appropriate to provide information on total dietary fibre.[35,36]

PROTEIN

As previously mentioned, all weight-control programmes entail a loss of approximately 15 % of lean mass, for which the diet must compensate.[37,38] Maintaining lean mass is important to sustain resting metabolism and energy expenditure, and to prevent a rebound effect after losing weight.[29,39–42]

The incorporation of increasing levels of protein and certain amino acids into these patients' treatment regimens is justified by several reasons, as reflected in Figure 4.[40,41,43]

Studies have shown that weight loss in patients fed high-protein diets is similar to that observed in those on a low-protein diet, despite the ingestion of more calories by the former group.[41,44] Similar results have been reported in other studies, which also described reduced loss of lean mass.[43,45,46] These results contrast with those of human studies, which reported that protein levels in isocaloric diets had no effect on satiety, hunger, satiation, weight loss, or cardiovascular health-related parameters.[8] Cats are the exception: high

Figure 4. From left to right: histidine, leucine, and serine molecules (petarg, Shutterstock.com).

Nutritional characteristics of protein and amino acids that are beneficial for weight loss:
- Low energy density (compared to fat).
- Low utilisation efficiency (0.55–0.65).
- Thermogenic effect.

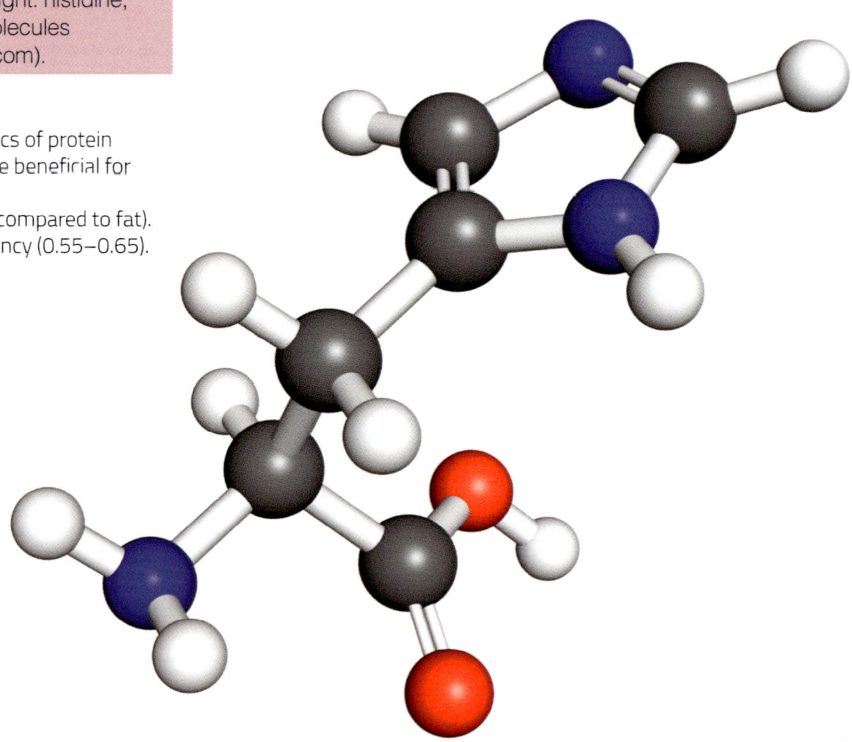

levels of protein in cat food are justified since cats are strict carnivores, and preferably use proteins and fats as energy sources.[47–49]

For dogs and cats, respectively, the daily protein allowance recommended by the NRC is 4.96 g/kg$^{0.67}$ or 3.28 g/kg$^{0.75}$, and the recommended crude protein (CP) content in foods is 25 and 50 g/1,000 kcal ME.[11] It must be remembered that the protein provided should be easily digestible, and of high quality and biological value. It seems advisable to increase these levels, in view of the loss of lean mass that occurs as part of any weight-loss programme.[37,38,43] We must ensure that patients receive this amount of protein, taking into account their reduced energy intake. Therefore, a minimum increase of 90 % over the protein allowance recommended by the NRC ensures that protein requirements are covered when the animal receives only 60 % of their daily maintenance requirements. Accordingly, 47.5 and 95.1 g CP/1,000 kcal ME are the minimum values for dogs and cats, respectively.

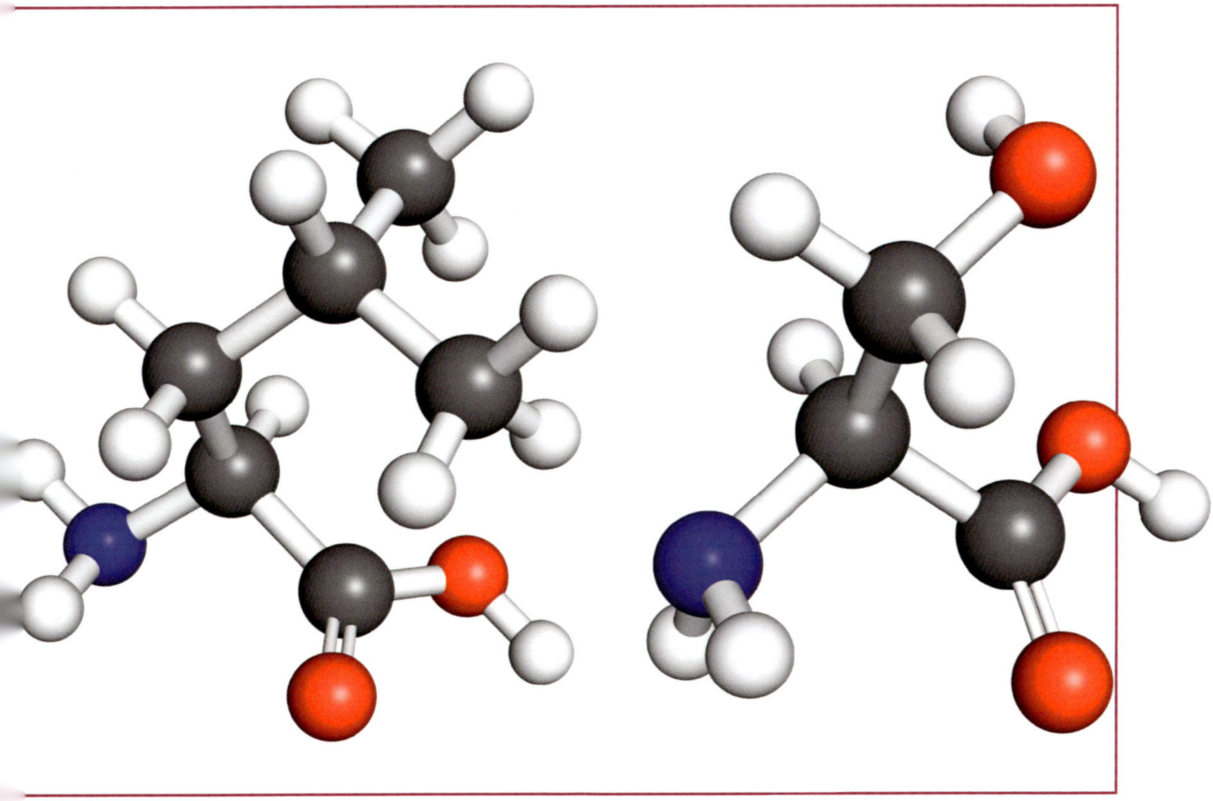

Example

Maléfico (Fig. 5) is an obese cat whose ideal weight is 6 kg, and would require 18.9 g CP/day (4.96 g CP × 6 kg$^{0.67}$× 1.15).

If the restricted diet covers 60 % of daily maintenance requirements, this would equate to 199.3 kcal ME/day (60 % × 100 kcal × 6 kg$^{0.67}$).

The label indicates that the product contains 22 % protein (220 g) and 3,875 kcal ME/kg DM. Therefore, this food does not cover the daily protein requirements:

199.3 × 220/3.875 = 11.31 g CP.

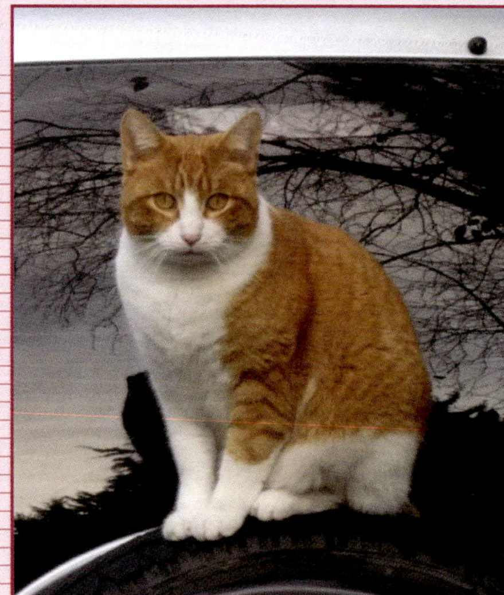

Figure 5. The ideal weight of *Maléfico* would be 6 kg.

For this diet to be suitable for our cat, it should provide the same level of energy, but have a 67.5 % higher protein content (36.85 %):

199.3 × 368.5/3.875 = 18.9 g of protein.

Most commercial food manufacturers (including some certified by FEDIAF and AAFCO) provide maintenance levels of protein per unit of energy that are somewhat higher than those recommended by the NRC. This could be due to differences in the origin and quality of the protein source, or possible losses that occur during the manufacturing process. The same applies to prescription diets for obese patients, in which protein levels are approximately 70 % greater than those recommended (for obese patients) by the NRC. Minimum values of 60 and 90 g CP/1,000 kcal ME are proposed for obese dogs and cats, respectively.

CARBOHYDRATES

As for healthy patients, there are no clear recommendations regarding the levels of this nutrient for obese pets. One of the myths in the area of nutrition is that hydrates predispose the individual to obesity and their absence in the diet promotes weight loss: the ingestion of energy, not the ingestion of carbohydrates, is associated with obesity. Nonetheless, it appears that the type of carbohydrate can affect levels of certain hormones (e.g. insulin, leptin, and ghrelin) involved in the regulation of energy homeostasis in the medium and long term.[50] Some authors recommend the use of certain types of carbohydrates (mainly cereals, which are the primary ingredient in pet foods) and their inclusion in diets owing to their effects on the control of satiety, blood glucose, insulin, and lipids.[51–53] However, the data are inconclusive.

In human medicine, as also observed in studies of dietary protein and fat, no significant differences in weight loss, or in any other parameters evaluated, were observed between patients on diets that were high or low in carbohydrates.[8] These data contrast with results obtained in cats.[53] It is advisable, especially in diabetic and obese cats, to maintain low levels of this nutrient and to preferably choose cereals with a low glycaemic index. The following are classified in order of increasing glycaemic index:

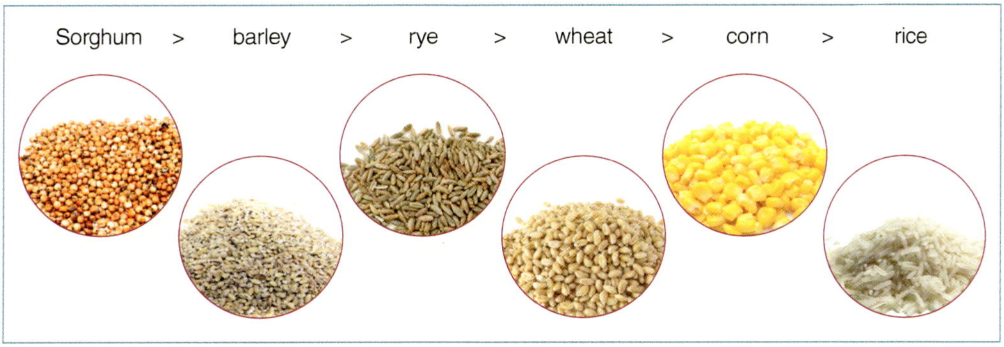

Although no veterinary studies have been conducted, research in human patients indicates that the inclusion of fructose leads to an increase in intra-abdominal fat, liver lipogenesis, and LDL cholesterol, and a decrease in insulin sensitivity and tolerance to glucose.[51,55,56] In the absence of relevant veterinary data, caution is recommended when incorporating products containing over 25 % of fructose-derived energy into the diets of obese patients.

As discussed above, there are no specific carbohydrate requirements for dogs or cats. However, there are specific tissues and situations that require mandatory provision of glucose: the central nervous system, red blood cells, lens, and retina; and periods of growth, lactation, and gestation. Therefore, the inclusion in the diet of a minimum of 50–62.5 g of carbohydrates/1,000 kcal ME is recommended.[11] According to food producers, for dogs this amount can be increased to 85–135 g. In the case of cats, it is important to adhere to the values recommended by the NRC.

DIETARY SUPPLEMENTS

The use of certain dietary supplements in weight-loss programmes appears to have few, if any, beneficial effects,[57] although protective effects against hepatic lipidosis during fasting have been described in cats.[56] Few peer-reviewed studies have demonstrated any benefits. Studies of the effects of substances such as L-carnitine,[59,60] soya isoflavones,[61] pyruvic acid,[62] vitamin A,[63] conjugated linoleic acid,[64,65] and diacylglycerols[66,67] remain inconclusive, owing to small sample sizes and inadequate trial durations.

Depending on the country, regulations governing these products may vary, or may not exist. For example, the EU authorised the use of L-carnitine in April 2015.[68]

By way of summary, Table 1 provides information on the recommended characteristics of foods for obese patients.

Table 1. Characteristics of food for obese patients.	
Nutrients	**Recommended amounts**
Energy (kcal ME/kg DM)	≤3,400
Fat (g) *	20–50
EPA DHA (g) *	>0.17
Vitamin E and Se (mg) *	0.6–1.2; 0.125
Fibre (g) *	35–60
Protein (g)*	>50 (dogs) and >100 (cats)
Carbohydrates (g) *	≥50 (up to 135 in dogs)

*Nutrient units/1,000 kcal ME

In reality, there is no ideal diet for these patients. The nutritional profile should be defined by the veterinary surgeon based on the individual history of each patient, their weight/body condition at the beginning of the programme, and the sociocultural environment of their owners. The different results obtained with weight-loss programmes suggest that, regardless of the type of diet, most diets provide a successful outcome in the long term provided they are approached with the necessary enthusiasm and persistence.

6 Dietary management in weight-loss programmes

Protocol

INTRODUCTION

In this chapter we will explain how a weight-loss programme should work. The programme should take into account the patient's requirements, the type of food, and the amount to be provided daily.

One practice that some people resort to is voluntary fasting for a few days. This practice is unacceptable in veterinary medicine and is particularly dangerous in cats owing to the risk of hepatic lipidosis.[1]

Fasting causes a series of changes in nutrient metabolism and body composition, both of which vary over time.[2,3] The main objective of these changes is to produce energy and maintain glycaemia in the vital organs. Table 1 summarises some of the changes that fasting causes in healthy animals.

As shown in Table 1, the first week of fasting constitutes an adaptation phase, during which carbohydrates are consumed first. This phase is relatively short in cats. After this transition period, energy and glucose are obtained from protein and fat. By the third or fourth week of fasting, marked decreases in fat reserves (approximately 50 %) and protein levels (25–30 %) are observed. To ensure that the patient can adequately recover, the decrease in muscle mass should not exceed 25–30 %. We can evaluate this situation using a blood test to measure levels of leukocytes, total proteins, albumin, and creatine kinase.[4–6]

Table 1. Changes during fasting in a healthy animal.

Days	Start	Duration	Nutrient	Metabolic pathway	Substrate	Organ
0–7	3 hours	12–28 hours	Carbohydrate	Glycogenolysis *	Glycogen	Liver
	4 hours	Variable	Fat	Gluconeogenesis	Glycerol	Liver and kidneys
	4 hours	Variable	Protein	Gluconeogenesis	Amino acids	Liver and kidneys
	48 hours	Variable	Fat	Oxidation	Fatty acids	Liver
0–3	Decrease in metabolism due to endocrine changes: decreases in thyroxine (T_4), triiodothyronine (T_3), and insulin					
5	The decrease in insulin increases lipolysis					

* In cats this pathway is associated with poor efficacy: concentrations of hepatic glucokinase and glycogen synthase are 10 times lower.

It is important to remember that fasting is a risky procedure in cats. Cats continuously use proteins as a source of energy and for the production of glucose, have a limited capacity to retain and conserve nitrogen and essential amino acids, and have high levels of endogenous urinary nitrogen excretion. Moreover, protein metabolism (catabolism, urea cycle, and gluconeogenesis) in cats does not adapt well to a lack of protein.[7]

It should be borne in mind that weight-loss programmes result in an inevitable reduction in muscle mass, the extent of which should not exceed 10–25 % of the total weight lost.[8] In cats, this loss of muscle mass can be masked by a less marked loss of fatty tissue.

This loss of lean mass equates to a decrease in maintenance requirements. Therefore, when establishing a weight-control programme, the loss of lean mass should be considered in order to recalculate the maintenance requirements and appropriately readjust the patient's caloric intake.

Human studies have shown that a weekly decrease of more than 2 % in body weight results in a marked loss of non-fatty tissue. As such, 2 % is considered a healthy limit.[9,10] A key advantage of this approach is that weight is lost rapidly, thereby motivating the patient (or in our case, the pet owner). However, there is little information available on the loss of non-fatty tissue in pets, and programmes that result in a weekly weight loss of a maximum of 3 % of body weight are common in dogs.

The use of highly restrictive programmes (dietary restriction >50 %), which quickly provide owners with evident results, can have the following effects:[11]

- Hunger-induced behavioural changes (e.g. hyperactivity, begging for and/or stealing food or consuming garbage) (Fig. 1).
- Excessive loss of muscle mass, which is exacerbated by the physical inactivity of obese patients.
- A rebound effect once the target weight has been reached.

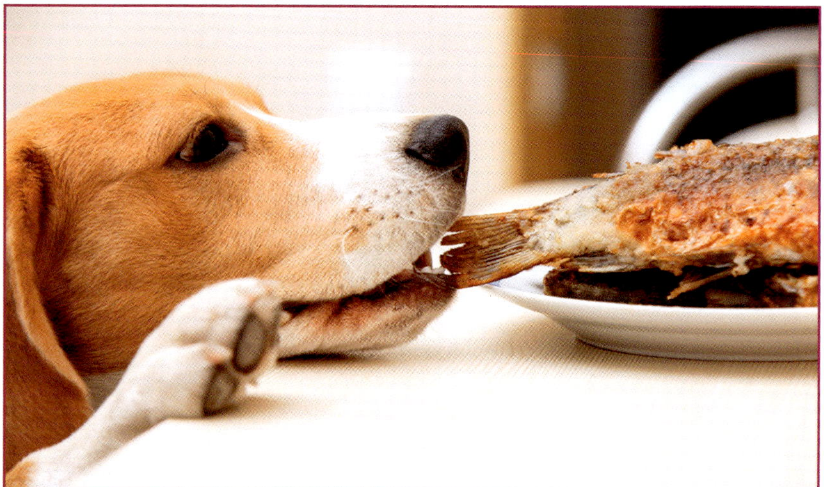

Figure 1. In some animals an overly restrictive diet can result in behavioural changes (e.g. stealing of food from the table) (Soloviova Liudmyla, Shutterstock.com).

Veterinary studies conducted over more than 40 years show that weight loss can vary considerably. In dogs, weight loss can vary depending on the severity of obesity (on a scale of 1–9), the extent and duration of dietary restriction, and the patient's sex (Fig. 2). To obtain the same outcome as in males, females require dietary restrictions of an additional 10 percentage points.[12,13] Thus, in the case of a dog with a BCS of 8/9, dietary restrictions of 25 % and 35 % would be applied to males and females, respectively. Weekly losses ranging from 0.7 % to 4.25 % have been reported in animals subjected to dietary restrictions of 40–60 % over periods of 7–28 weeks, independent of sex. Similar outcomes have been reported in cats: weekly losses range from 0.4–1.5 %, depending on the level of restriction (25–50 %).

Therefore, the optimal weekly weight loss is 1–3 % in dogs and 1–1.5 % in cats.[4-17] Any weight loss (e.g. 0.5 %) is welcome news to the owner and the veterinary team, although it should be borne in mind that a lower rate of weight loss implies prolonged dietary restriction. In our programmes, we typically establish a weekly weight-loss goal of 1.5 %, and actual losses range from 0.9–1.3 %.

The first step in any weight-loss programme is to determine the patient's requirements. Next, the type of food is selected and the recommended daily amount established.

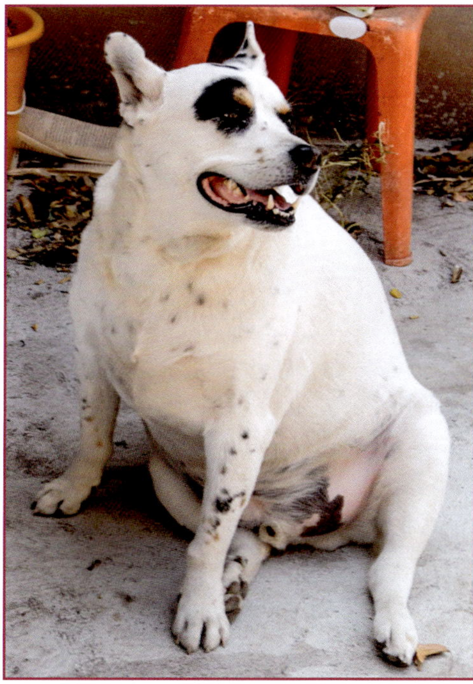

Figure 2. In dogs, dietary restrictions vary depending on sex (Sitthipong Pengjan, Shutterstock.com).

HOW ARE THE PATIENT'S REQUIREMENTS DETERMINED?

There are several ways to calculate a patient's energy requirements. In the past, weight-loss programmes were designed by establishing dietary restrictions based on the target (or ideal) weight. Currently, two main approaches are used: programmes that establish restrictions based on current weight (overweight or obese patients); and programmes that are based on a target weight. The choice of approach depends on the experience of the veterinary surgeon, the degree of overweight, and the duration of overweight/obesity.

Energy requirements

Before we begin, we will briefly summarise the body's energy requirements:

- **Basal metabolism (BM):** minimum energy requirements of an animal that is at complete rest and does not ingest food.
- **Basal metabolism at rest (BMR):** energy requirements of an animal that is at rest and ingests food (**resting energy requirement or RER**); energy is produced in the form of heat generated by thermal increases (digestive and metabolic processes) and the activity of the autonomic nervous system. The BMR mainly covers the requirements of lean tissue, since fatty tissue is inert from the metabolic point of view.
- **Maintenance energy requirement (MER):** energy required to ensure an energy balance of zero, considering activity and thermoregulation. The MER is 70–75 % higher than the BMR.[18,19]

Target weight and RER

Here, we will calculate the RER based on the optimal (target) weight of the patient. The RER is calculated using the following equations:

Equation 1	$RER\ (kcal/day) = 70 \times Body\ weight^{0.75}\ (kg)$

Equation 2	$RER\ (kcal/day) = 30 \times Body\ weight\ (kg) + 70$

Equation 1 can be used for patients of any weight, while Equation 2 is used for those weighing 2–25 kg. Both equations produce similar results in the weight range of 4–25 kg and for a BCS ≥7/9. Outside this range the results obtained can vary by up to 8 %.

In the case of dogs, the result of these equations represents a mean of 54 % of the maintenance energy requirements proposed by the National Research Council (NRC) in 2006 using the following equation:

Equation 3	$MER_{dogs}\ (kcal/day) = 130 \times Body\ weight^{0.75}\ (kg)$

When we analyse the variation in weekly weight loss, we find that in the body weight range of 2.5–50 kg the weekly weight loss calculated exceeds the recommended 1.5 % per week: minimum values of 1.6 % are obtained for the highest weights, and as body weight decreases values reach 3–3.5 % (e.g. for a 5-kg dog with a BCS of 7/9, the weekly loss calculated would be 3.3 %; for a 50-kg dog with a BCS of 7/9 the corresponding value would be 1.6 %). Variations in weekly weight loss are inversely correlated with the percentage of overweight. Thus, lower values are obtained for dogs with a BCS of 9/9.

In cats, the result of both equations (1 and 2) equates to 77 % of the MER proposed by the NRC (2006) with the following equation:

Equation 4	MER_{cats} (kcal/day) = 100 × Body weight$^{0.67}$ (kg)

Analysis of weekly weight loss reveals a more conservative progression (mean value, 1 %).

Example 1

Dog with a current weight of 14 kg (e.g. Cocker Spaniel), a BCS of 8/9, 30 % overweight, and a target weight of 10.8 kg.

Applying Equation 1:

RER (kcal/day) = 70 × Body weight$^{0.75}$

RER (kcal/day) = 70 × 10.8$^{0.75}$

RER (kcal/day) = 416.14

If we calculate the weekly losses and the restriction of MER, we obtain values of 2.4 % and 54 %, respectively (calculations are shown in subsequent examples). This is a more aggressive regimen than that proposed by NRC recommendations.

Example 2

Cat with a current weight of 7.5 kg (e.g. domestic shorthair cat), a BCS of 8/9, 30 % overweight, and a target weight of 5.77 kg.

Applying Equation 1:

RER (kcal/day) = 70 × Body weight$^{0.75}$

RER (kcal/day) = 70 × 5.77$^{0.75}$

RER (kcal/day) = 260.6

In this case, the equation proposes a weekly loss and MER restriction of 0.9 % and 80 %, respectively. These values are more conservative than those obtained using the NRC recommendations, and correspond to a weekly weight loss of less than the 1.5 % target.

By subtracting daily mass loss from current weight

In this case, MER is determined based on the current weight of the obese patient. To this end, we can use Equations 1 and 2, applying a correction factor of 1.4 for dogs and 1.2–1.4 for cats.[20–22]

As a rule of thumb it is assumed that each gram of weight lost equates to 7.728 kcal of energy.

The next step is to establish the target weekly weight loss. Next, the loss in energy corresponding to the expected daily mass loss should be calculated, assuming an energy density comparable to that of fat.

This assumption is based on the fact that lost weight consists of 87 % fat, fluids, glycogen, and protein. This is a widely accepted simplification made to facilitate calculations.[8,23,24]

With this method, the calculations obtained are valid throughout the entire body weight range (2.5–60 kg) and for all BCS values in both dogs and cats. The RER for a weekly loss of 1.5 %, according to Equations 1 and 2, is reduced to 67 % and 74 % for dogs and cats, respectively.

This is an effective prediction method, but is somewhat unwieldy for use in routine practice.

In cats a specific equation for overweight animals (BCS >5/9) is used:

Equation 5	$MER_{obese\ cats}$ (kcal/day) = 130 (kcal) × Body weight$^{0.4}$ (kg)

This equation is not practical for use in clinical practice. It is easier to estimate the target weight and apply Equation 4 and the corresponding correction factor. The differences between the 2 equations are negligible for a BCS >8/9. For lower scores Equation 5 is 9–10 % more restrictive.

Example 3

Dog with a current weight of 14 kg (e.g. Cocker Spaniel), a BCS of 8/9, 30 % overweight, and weekly weight loss target of 1.5 %.

Applying Equation 1 with a correction factor of 1.4:

MER (kcal/day) = 1.4 × (70 × Body weight$^{0.75}$)

MER (kcal/day) = 1.4 × (70 × 14$^{0.75}$)

MER (kcal/day) = 709.3

Weekly weight loss = 14 kg × 1.5 %; Weekly weight loss = 210 g

Energy content of daily weight loss = (210 g × 7.728 kcal/g)/7

Energy content of daily weight loss = 231.8 kcal

MER_{day} = MER - Energy content of daily weight loss; MER_{day} = 477.45 kcal/day

In this case the MER is reduced to 67 % to achieve a weight loss of 1.5 %.

Example 4

Cat with a current weight of 7.5 kg (e.g. domestic shorthair), a BCS of 8/9, 30 % overweight, and a weekly weight loss target of 1.5 %.

Applying Equation 1 with a correction factor of 1.4:

MER (kcal/day) = 1.4 × (70 × Body weight$^{0.75}$)

MER (kcal/day) = 1.4 × (70 × 7.5$^{0.75}$)

MER (kcal/day) = 444.14

Weekly weight loss = 7.5 kg × 1.5 %; Weekly weight loss = 113 g

Energy content of daily weight loss = (113 g × 7.728 kcal/g)/7

Energy content of daily weight loss = 124.2 kcal

MER_{day} = MER - Energy content of daily weight loss; MER_{day} = 319.9 kcal/day

In this case the MER is reduced to 72 % to achieve a weight loss of 1.5 %.

Dietary restriction based on an optimal (target) weight considering maintenance requirements

This approach constitutes a combination of the two aforementioned methods. In this case, Equations 3 and 4 are used, and a correction factor applied. For a weekly loss of 1.5 % of current body weight, the MER is reduced to 70 % (dogs) or 60 % (cats). Depending on the criterion of the veterinary surgeon and the patient's comorbidities, the MER in dogs can be reduced to a maximum of 50 % (this value equates to a weekly weight loss of approximately 2.5 %).

In the case of cats it is crucial to remember that caloric restriction should ensure that the animal is provided with at least 70 % of its RER or 60 % of its MER, given the risk of developing hepatic lipidosis. To ensure no risk to health, the upper limit of the weekly weight loss should be 1.5 %, although preferably this should be adjusted to 1 % (75 % of MER).

As a rule of thumb, we can establish a margin of safety by aiming for an energy contribution of 50–60 % of the MER.

This is a simple system, in our opinion, that uses equations to determine maintenance energy requirements in dogs and cats, independent of their level of activity (e.g. sporting animals), physiological stage (e.g. lactation), or diseases (e.g. obesity, chronic disease). In any of these three situations, the MER will be modified (e.g. in a lactating animal MER may be multiplied by 3).

Example 5

Dog with a current weight of 14 kg (e.g. Cocker Spaniel), a BCS of 8/9, 30 % overweight, a weekly weight loss of 1.5 %, and a target weight of 10.8 kg.

Applying Equation 3 with a 70 % restriction:

$MER_{dogs} = 130 \times \text{Body weight}^{0.75}$

$MER_{day} = 70\ \% \times (130 \times 10.8^{0.75})$; $MER_{day} = 541$ kcal/day

If the clinician considers that owing to the presence of other processes (e.g. orthopaedic disease) the patient should aim for a weekly weight loss of 2 %, the MER is reduced to less than 60 %.

Example 6

Cat with a current weight of 7.5 kg (e.g. domestic shorthair), a BCS of 8/9, 30 % overweight, a weekly weight loss of 1.5 %, and a target weight of 5.77 kg.

Applying Equation 4 with a 60 % restriction:

$MER_{cats} = 100 \times \text{Body weight}^{0.67}$

$MER_{day} = 60\ \% \times (100 \times 5.77^{0.67})$; $MER_{day} = 194.13$ kcal/day

WHAT IS THE PATIENT'S DAILY RATION?

Once the appropriate prescription food has been selected in accordance with the patient's requirements, the next step is to determine the amount of food the patient should receive. The characteristics of different nutrients and their incorporation into the body have already been discussed in the chapter on prescription foods.

In the case of commercial foods, this calculation can be performed in two ways: using the information provided on the product label, or based on the energy content of the food. Finally, based on the patient's energy requirements and the energy content of the food, the recommended daily amount can be calculated.

Calculation based on product label information

This is the simplest approach for the veterinary surgeon, but also the least professional. The recommended daily amount is indicated in the product information provided by pet food manufacturers on the product label, in the technical information provided on the packet, or on the corresponding web page (which may also recommend specific dietary programmes). From our point of view, this approach suffers from several limitations:

- It allows owners to make decisions, which are sometimes erroneous, based on the information provided on the packet. This in turn:
  - Increases the pet owner's lack of conviction about their pet's condition.
  - Decreases trust in the veterinary surgeon.
  - Promotes substitution of one product with another without considering their respective characteristics. For example, analysis of the stated composition of certain prescription foods has revealed variations of ±10–30 % in energy content between similar products of different brands.

- Underestimates the patient's BCS and target weight. As also observed in human medicine, when asked to indicate their pet's BCS using an evaluation chart owners tend to select 1 point less than the true score.
- The daily recommendations provided on the product label are generally calculated for a relatively broad weight range.

- The work of the veterinary surgeon is devalued.
- Pet owners are not provided with a personalised consultation.
- The calculations may vary depending on the methodology used by the manufacturer.

Calculation based on the energy content of the food

This approach allows determination of the metabolisable energy (ME) based on the information provided by the manufacturer or calculation of the energy content of the nutrients of the food, whether commercial or prepared at home.

There are two ways of calculating ME:[18,19]

- The equations proposed by the NRC (2006). The ME of a food depends on the gross energy, the digestibility of the energy, the digestible energy, the crude fibre or total dietary fibre content, and the energy lost via urine. The complex formulas used allow accurate estimation of the ME of most commercial foods, since they include a correction factor for fibre (provided that the crude fibre content, expressed as a percentage of dry matter, does not exceed 8 %).
- The modified Atwater equation. This equation provides a generic means of predicting the approximate ME content of a pet food based on the energy of the nutrients. According to this equation, the number of calories provided by each nutrient type is as follows: crude protein (CP), 3.5 kcal/g; crude fat (CF), 8.5 kcal/g; carbohydrates (nitrogen-free extracts or NFE), 3.5 kcal/g.

Equation 6	$\text{ME (kcal)} = (\text{g CP} \times 3.5\ \text{kcal}) + (\text{g CF} \times 8.5\ \text{kcal}) + (\text{g NFE} \times 3.5\ \text{kcal})$

This equation underestimates the ME of homemade foods and of some highly digestible commercially available foods. However, it is an easy calculation and its use is widespread (e.g. FEDIAF and AAFCO).

Example 7

Determine the ME content of dog food with the following composition: 30 % raw protein, 8.8 % raw fat, and 33.2 % carbohydrates.

Applying Equation 6:

ME (kcal) = (g CP × 3.5 kcal) + (g CF × 8.5 kcal) + (g NFE × 3.5 kcal)

ME (kcal/100 g) = (30 × 3.5) + (8.8 × 8.5) + (33.2 × 3.5)

ME (kcal/100 g) = 296 kcal

Now that we know the energy content of the food, the next step in the weight-loss programme is to determine the total recommended daily amount. This is simply a question of correlating the MER with the ME of the selected food.

Recommended daily amount = MER/ME

Continuing with Example 5 and the characteristics of the food described above:

MER_{day} = 541 kcal/day; ME = 296 kcal/100 g

Recommended daily amount (g) = (541 × 100)/296 = 182.8 g/day

HOW IS THE RECOMMENDED DAILY RATION ADMINISTERED TO THE PATIENT?

Once we have determined the amount of food our patient should receive, we must reach an agreement with the owner on the best means of administering it. As mentioned above, the participation of pet owners in the decision-making process is key to ensuring successful pet nutrition: we should not attempt to force our opinion on the pet owner unless absolutely necessary, but instead should seek their cooperation. This is all the more important where sick pets are concerned.

In the case of healthy animals, three main feeding options are considered: ad libitum, restricted ad libitum, and fixed-schedule controlled feeding.

Many obese patients exhibit behavioural alterations that result in erratic feeding behaviour (mediated by secondary pathways and by serotonin and related neurotransmitters). Given this phenomenon, and taking into account the mechanisms that control satiety, it is advisable to divide the recommended daily amount into several portions offered throughout the day, i.e. **fixed-schedule controlled feeding**. The objective is to provide the animal with a diet that corresponds to their requirements and to modify the bad habits that have developed in the owner-pet relationship.

The total daily ration is administered in several portions, and the animal's access to each portion is limited to 10–20 minutes, or 1–2 hours in the case of some cats (Fig. 3). Pets are alerted in advance of the meal, which should always be consumed in the same location (e.g. patio, kitchen, laundry room). Once the allocated time has passed, the plate is removed and no more food provided until the next sitting. Surplus food should not be incorporated into the subsequent ration, with two exceptions:

- Some dogs and cats, when provided with their ration in three portions, do not consume the same amounts in each sitting; in this case the amount of food provided in the evening can be reduced, and that provided in the other two portions increased (e.g. 40 %:40 %:20 %).
- As mentioned above, care should be taken when reducing the food intake of cats.

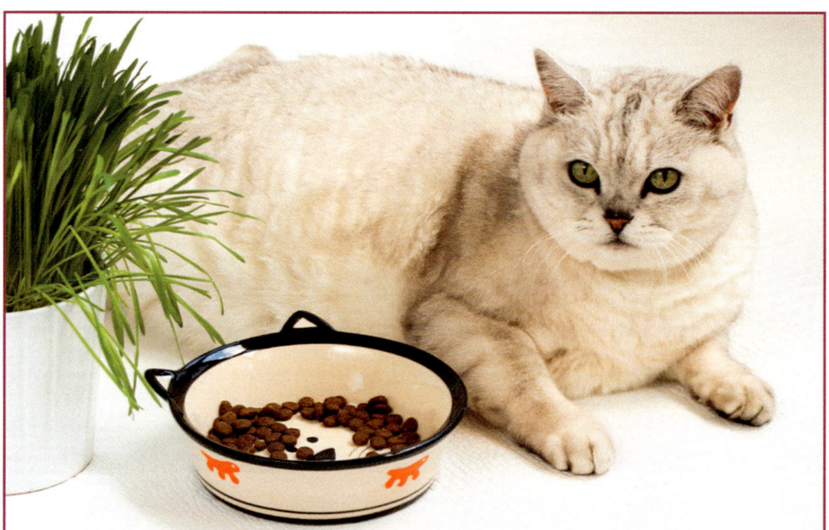

Figure 3. Some cats require access for several hours to each portion of their daily ration (Svetlana.Is, Shutterstock.com).

The number of times a pet should eat to obtain the best results is unknown. Given the personal and professional obligations of most pet owners, we generally propose that they offer the daily ration in 2 or 3 portions at intervals of 8–10 hours. However, as noted above, the satiety pattern can vary considerably between animals.

In the case of cats, **restricted ad libitum** feeding may be a good option, since cats tend to consume small portions throughout the day independent of their circadian rhythm. The daily ration is calculated based on the requirements of the pet and is administered onto their plate or via a dispenser until it has been fully consumed. Unfortunately, this approach is only feasible in single-animal homes.

There are a number of additional general recommendations that are worth remembering:

- Be precise in calculating the daily ration. Use a scales to measure the daily ration in grams. Do not use alternative units such as cups or measuring spoons (differences can reach up to 20 % depending on particle size) (Fig. 4).
- Try to ensure that the pet's daily ration can be easily divided into multiple portions by the owner. As mentioned above, all meals need not be identical in size.

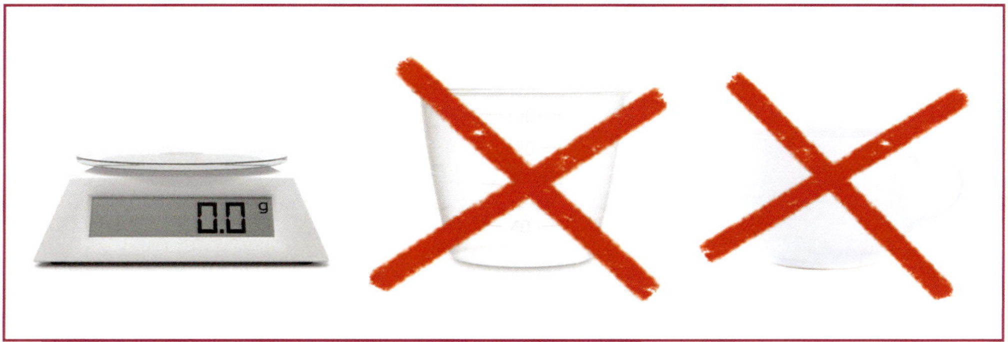

Figure 4. It is essential to weigh the food to accurately measure the amount that the animal must ingest daily (Fedorov Ivan Sergeevich/Coprid/skynetphoto, Shutterstock.com).

- In houses with several animals, each should have their own dish and a separate, quiet place to eat (to avoid competition). Commercially available automated feeders allow remote control of a variety of parameters, including quantity, time of administration, and duration of availability, and can be very useful in these cases (Fig. 5).

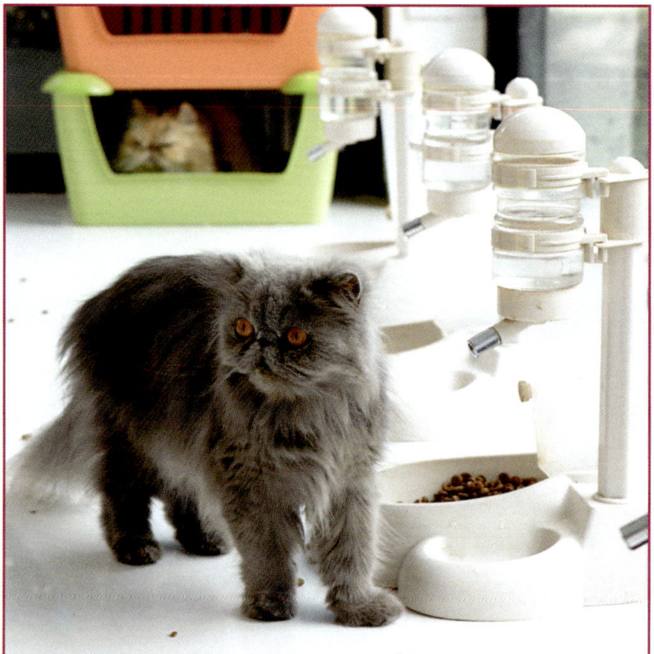

Figure 5. Automated water and food dispensers (Zoo Design, Shutterstock.com).

Table 2. Weight (kg) corresponding to the desired percentage of weight to be lost.

Week	1 %	1.5 %
0	7.50	7.50
1	7.43	7.39
2	7.35	7.28
3	7.28	7.17
4	7.20	7.06
5	7.13	6.95
6	7.06	6.85
7	6.99	6.75
8	6.92	6.65
9	6.85	6.55
10	6.78	6.45
11	6.72	6.35
12	6.65	6.26
13	6.58	6.16
14	6.52	5.98
15	6.45	5.80
16	6.39	
17	6.32	
18	6.26	
19	6.20	
20	6.13	
21	6.07	
22	6.01	
23	5.95	
24	5.89	

MONITORING PROGRESS

Regular monitoring of the patient is essential to ensure successful weight-loss. This allows quantification of the patient's weight loss and, perhaps more importantly, reinforces the efforts of the pet owner, thereby increasing their trust in the veterinary care team and their determination to ensure that their pet recovers (Fig. 6).

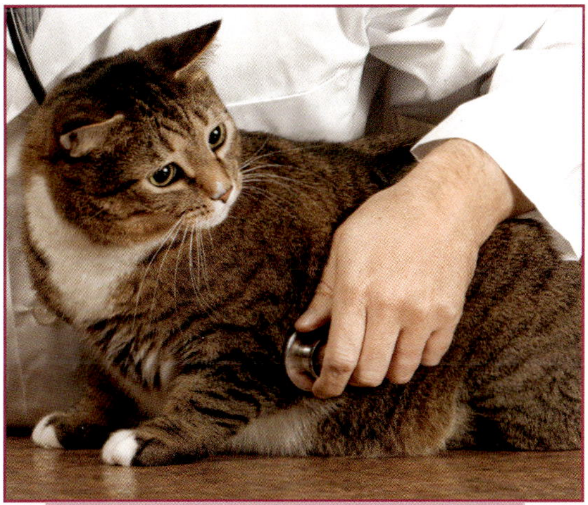

Figure 6. The owner must be convinced that their pet's obesity is a disease (Mr. Nikon, Shutterstock.com).

This will already have been discussed with the owner when initially proposing the weight-loss programme (duration and cost of treatment, expected weight loss, etc.).

As a rule, the first examination should take place 15–30 days after beginning the programme. Based on these findings, the programme should either be continued as is or adjusted as necessary. In the event that the weight loss does not correspond to the established target, the MER, and therefore the daily ration, should be increased or decreased by 10–15 %. The use of a prediction table (Table 2) and graph (Fig. 7) based on the duration of the treatment course can facilitate follow-up.

Weight-loss programmes are not static, nor based exclusively on calculations, which are used only to establish a treatment starting-point.

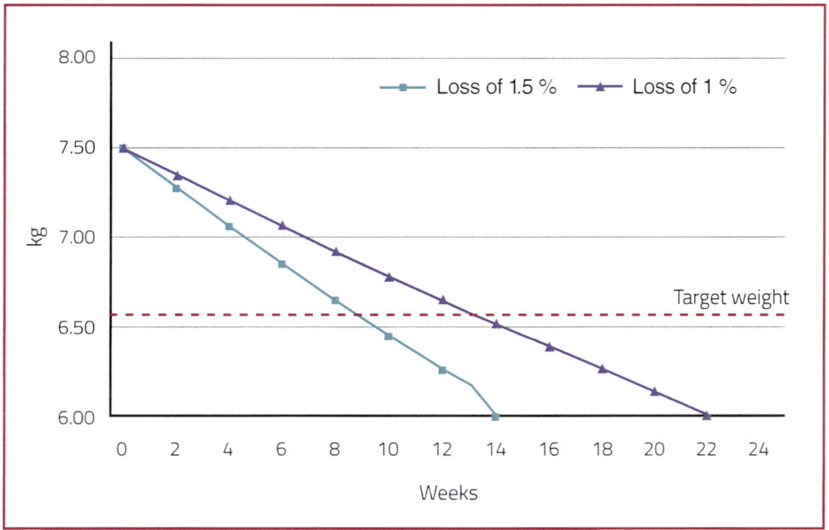

Figure 7. Graph corresponding to the data in Table 2.

7 Treatment of obesity

Workplan

INITIAL APPROACH

As soon as the owner indicates that they are ready to talk about the issue, it is time to explain the disease to them. The first step is to weigh and assess the BCS of the patient to establish the target weight.

There are two types of patients: those whose clinical history from an early age is already known; and new adult patients (Fig. 1). In the case of the former it will be necessary to analyse changes in weight and body conformation over time and determine their relative weight. This is the relationship between current weight and previous weight: a value >1 is indicative of disease. If the patient is new (Fig. 2) it will be necessary to record their weight and body condition in the medical record (this evaluation is described in Chapter 3). Body condition scoring and morphometric measurements are two simple and economical methods that can be used in clinical practice. The use of computer software (e.g. Excel) makes these tasks easier.

As with most diseases, it will be necessary to complete the study with routine blood tests (e.g. haematometry, biochemical analysis, lipid metabolism), endocrine profiles (e.g. determination of diabetic, thyroid, or adrenal disorders), analyses of specific parameters (e.g. leptin and adiponectin), and diagnostic imaging techniques (in particular liver ultrasound).

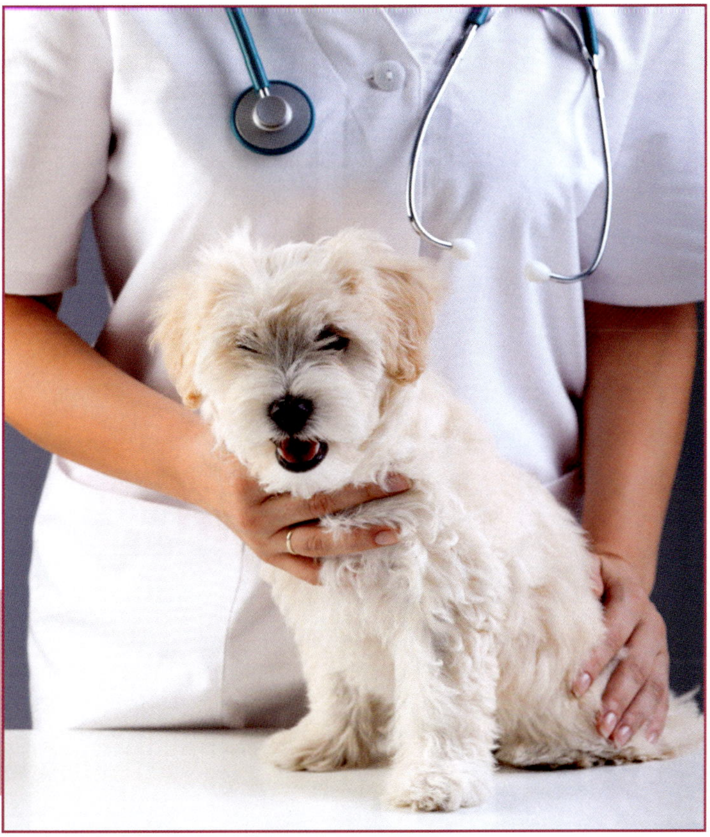

Figure 1. Follow-up of changes in weight and body conformation is easier in patients that have attended the clinic since they were puppies (Ilike, Shutterstock.com).

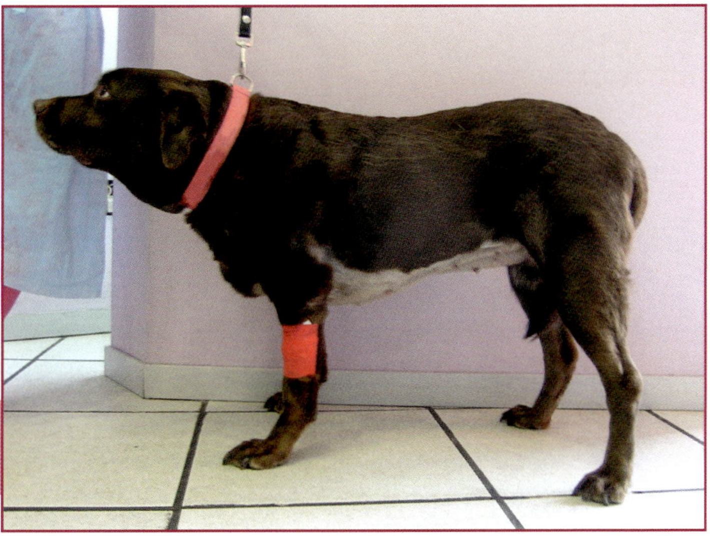

Figure 2. Patient after removal of several small lipomas.

Once the disease has been diagnosed, we can then attempt to connect with the owner at the emotional level in order to engender commitment and compliance. The following strategies can be used to motivate the owner:

- Compare the life expectancy of a healthy pet with that of an obese pet (Fig. 3).
- Have the owner put on a vest or a backpack containing a weight equivalent to the overweight of the pet. If the patient is 15 % overweight, add 15 % of the owner's weight (i.e. if they weigh 60 kg, place 9 kg in the backpack). They are unlikely to stand for more than 2 minutes while bearing this extra weight (Fig. 4).
- Provide examples of data from human studies so that the owner perceives the similarities between the treatment protocols. Reinforce the owner's empathy towards their pet's condition.
- Try to ensure that pet owners coincide in the waiting room with other owners whose pets have already started treatment programmes and have seen beneficial effects.

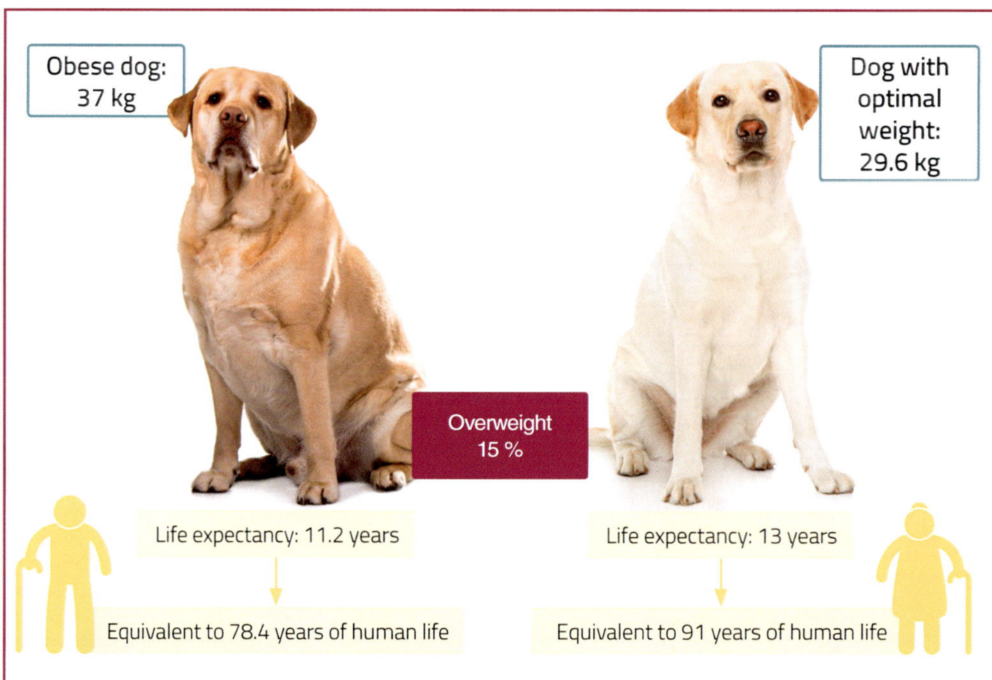
Obese dog: 37 kg
Dog with optimal weight: 29.6 kg
Overweight 15 %
Life expectancy: 11.2 years
Equivalent to 78.4 years of human life
Life expectancy: 13 years
Equivalent to 91 years of human life

Figure 3. Life expectancy in a dog with and without overweight (Sponner/Jagodka, Shutterstock.com).

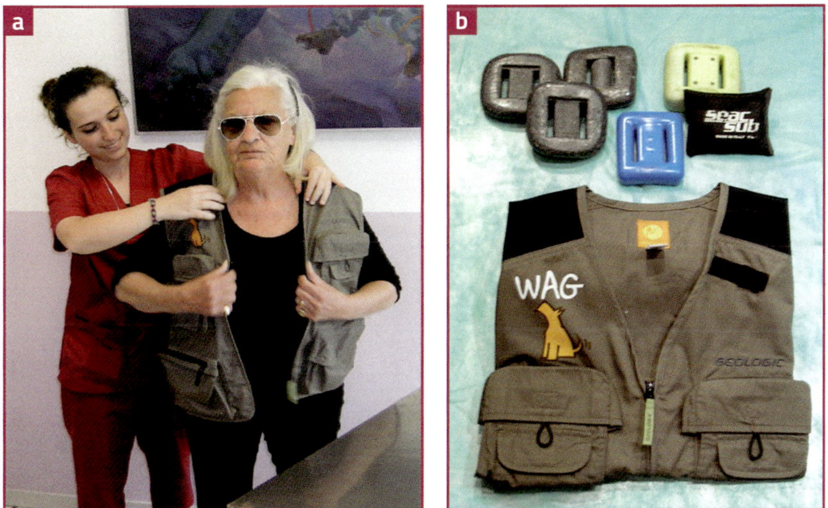

Figure 4. Client with weighted backpack to simulate the extra load borne by the overweight patient (a). Backpack and weights used (b).

- Take photographs at each of the follow-up examinations to show the owner during moments of doubt or show them images of patients who have reached their optimal weight (Figs. 5 and 6).
- Provide a basic bibliography on obesity and overweight.

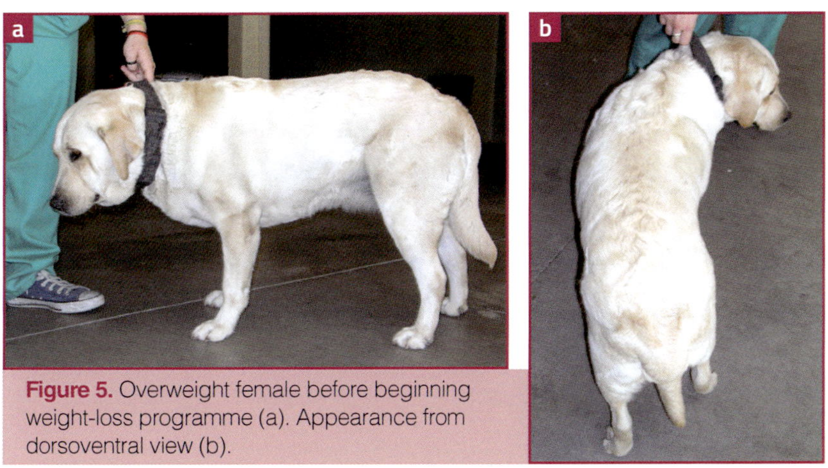

Figure 5. Overweight female before beginning weight-loss programme (a). Appearance from dorsoventral view (b).

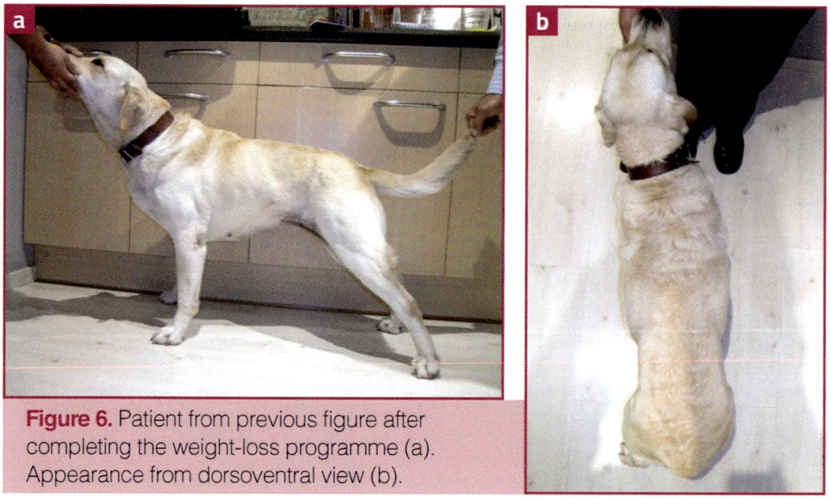

Figure 6. Patient from previous figure after completing the weight-loss programme (a). Appearance from dorsoventral view (b).

DURATION AND COST OF TREATMENT

Knowledge of the duration of the treatment and the total cost is one of the factors that will help encourage owner participation in the treatment programme.

The duration of the weight-loss programme is easy to calculate. Simply relate the total amount of weight that needs to be lost to the desired weekly weight loss.

Example

Misco (Fig. 7) is a mixed-breed dog with an initial weight of 14 kg, a BCS of 8/9, overweight of 30 %, with a weekly target weight loss of 1.5 %. This case was relatively straightforward, since the reason for the initial consultation was to resolve the patient's weight problem, and the family environment was health-oriented. The calculations were as follows:

- This patient had to lose 3.23 kg, which was the difference between the weight at the time of consultation and the ideal weight.
- This implied a weight loss of 0.21 kg/week (14 kg × 1.5 %).
- In this case, the duration was 15.4 weeks (3.23 kg/0.21 kg/week) (Fig. 8).

To determine the approximate cost of treatment, it will be necessary to include a fixed cost (covering the prescription diet), and different variable costs: pharmacological treatments, private facilities for exercise, professional consultations, and additional tests. These last two costs form part of the diagnosis, treatment, and prognosis of any disease.

Continuing with the previous example, and analysing the diet, we can determine the following:

- If the daily requirements are 541 kcal ME and the prescription food provides 296 kcal/100 g, the dog should consume 182.8 g/day.
- The consumption calculated for the period described would be: 182.8 g/day × 7 days/week × 15.4 weeks = 19.7 kg of food in total.
- The quantities in which the food can be purchased vary considerably (1.5–14 kg). It is advisable to examine the patient at 30 days. Therefore, our advice is to choose a quantity that can be adjusted to that period: 182.8 g × 30 days = 5.48 kg consumed.
- We recommend performing this calculation to avoid a large economic outlay, since this could result in cessation of the programme. Furthermore, owners of small- or medium-sized patients may prefer intermediate quantities to avoid spoilage.

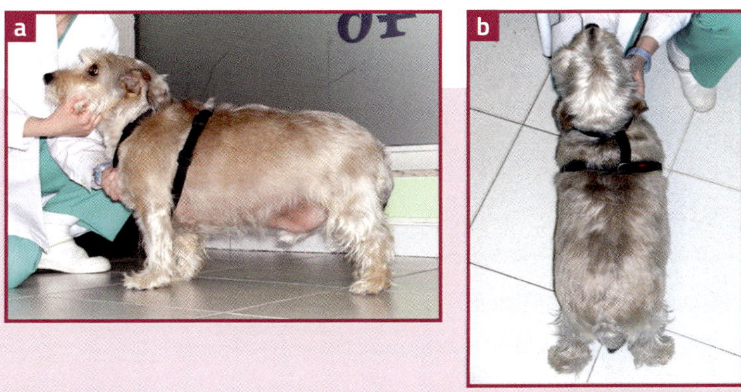

Figure 7. *Misco*, an overweight patient, before beginning a weight-loss programme (a). Appearance from dorsoventral view (b).

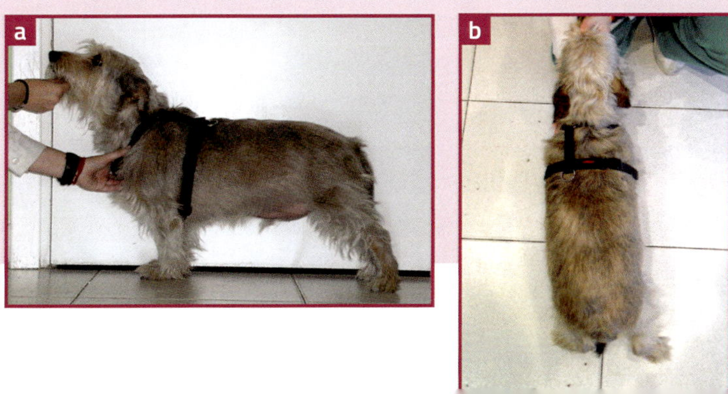

Figure 8. *Misco* at the end of the weight-loss programme (a). Appearance from dorsoventral view (b).

- The last step is to multiply the sale price to the public by the number of units the owner will need. Suppose the price is €5/kg: €19.7 kg × €5/kg = €98.53.
- To underscore the value of the treatment programme, simply divide the total cost by the number of days: €98.53/108 days = €0.91/day. In our opinion this is a reasonable cost for any responsible owner. It is also good to remind the owner of what Hippocrates said: "Let your medicine be your food, and food your medicine."

FOOD SELECTION

We have already discussed the recommended composition of prescription foods for our patients, as well as differences in the energy density of different foods.[1] Therefore, the first step is to compare foods by expressing their composition in units of nutrients (mg or g) per unit of metabolisable energy (kcal) and determine which best suits the needs of our patient.[2] Next, it is advisable to recommend the owners 3 or 4 different options that can be easily purchased.

In the pet food sector there are over 100 different brands that can be used for the treatment or prevention of overweight. The choice of one over another is at the discretion of the veterinary professional.

If we insist on prescribing a specific food that the owner has trouble acquiring (due to cost or accessibility), we are giving them an excuse to abandon the weight-loss programme.

AGREED REWARDS

A successful dietary treatment programme requires the owner to be flexible with their habits and customs. Most owners enjoy offering food to their animals as a sign of affection. The impact of such rewards on pet health is controversial; while some support the use of rewards, others feel that they may predispose animals to overweight.[3,4] The literature demonstrates the value of using rewards as a means of positive reinforcement. However, when formulating prescription diets it is prudent to substitute a small part of the ration with rewards, provided they do not exceed 10 % of the daily caloric needs.

The products used should be specific to the target species. Homemade food, especially those rich in fat or salt, should be avoided. If homemade food cannot be avoided, it should at least have a high moisture and protein content (Fig. 9).

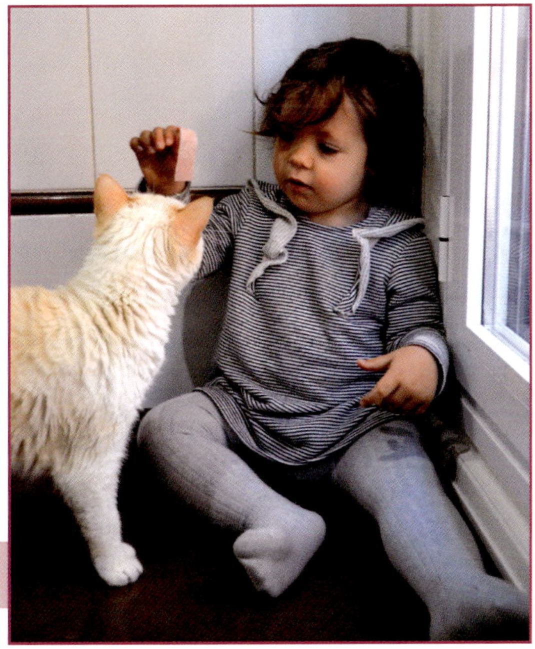

Figure 9. If homemade food is offered, it must have high water and protein content.

EXERCISE AND LIFESTYLE

As already discussed in Chapter 1, certain pet owner behaviours can significantly influence the development of disease. The first step is to try to modify these behaviours.

Establishing an exercise programme for the pet has three main objectives:

- Increase daily energy expenditure.
- Promote muscle tone: it should be borne in mind that age and sedentary lifestyle are associated with a loss of approximately 18–20 % of lean tissue and muscle atrophy.
- Create a bond with the pet.

Sport or exercise increase energy expenditure by reversing the energetic imbalance of the obese patient (zero energy balance). With each weekly hour of activity, regardless of type, the risk of obesity decreases.[5,6] Interestingly however, the results of some epidemiological surveys appear to contrast with the prevalence of the disease:

- Owners do not consider exercise important for their pets.[7]
- Almost 80 % say that they walk their pets.[8]
- According to surveys, 1 in 5 obese dogs exercise (walking, jogging, running, or swimming) accompanied by their owners: they walk/run for 2.5 hours per week (10 %) or swim for 15 minutes twice per week (3 %).
- On the other hand, the amount of exercise performed decreases with increasing age.[5]

The exercise performed by the vast majority of pets, especially dogs, has no significant effect on their daily energy requirements. There is some controversy regarding results obtained in companion animals. For example, one study found that swimming failed to improve weight loss in dogs: comparison of two groups of dieting dogs, one of which swam for 20 minutes twice per week, showed that mean weight loss was lower in the swimming group than the control group (10.3 % vs. 15.7 %), although loss of body fat was higher (16 % versus 7.5 %).[9] These results are surprising, as swimming appears to be associated with a high level of energy expenditure. In humans, 1 hour of swimming crawl style at a moderate pace equates to approximately 25 % of daily requirements, although this has not been quantified in animals. Moreover, the energy expended by dogs varies depending on the pectoral width of the breed.[10] While some authors have reported a positive effect of exercise (running or jogging) on weight loss (13.9 % vs. 12.9 %), these differences were not significant.[11]

The optimal amount of exercise to prevent overweight has not been determined. For a healthy animal to obtain a benefit from sports activities, the calories expended performing physical activity should ideally correspond to at least 5 % of daily requirements. Canids are athletes per se, and to reach this threshold would need to run (10 km/h) for 20–30 minutes, although this will vary depending on the size of a given breed (biomechanical effect).[10,12] Our observations indicate that the vast majority of dogs that live in large cities (e.g. Madrid) walk about 30–40 minutes per day (divided into three walks), covering a distance of approximately 3 km. This qualifies as low-level exercise (Fig. 10).

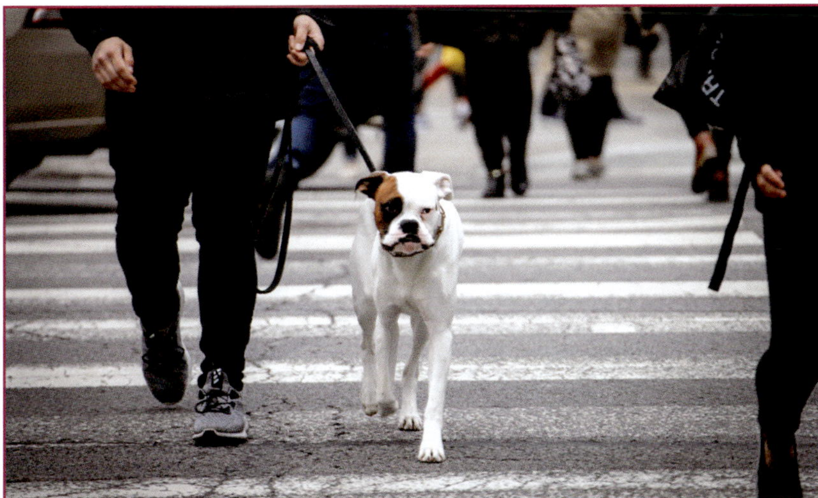

Figure 10. Normal walks around the city do not provide sufficient exercise to prevent overweight (jodrum, Shutterstock.com).

Moderate activity for 15–30 minutes per day, at least 5 days per week, is the minimum required and poses little risk to health.[14]

Based on calculations of the energy deficit per unit of weight lost, an overweight dog (BCS, 7/9) should walk 15 km per day in order to consume the energy corresponding to 50 % of the estimated weight loss (weekly weight loss of 1.5 %). Great care should be taken since these patients are typically over 6 years of age, sedentary, and have cardiovascular compromise or orthopaedic limitations[13] (Fig. 11). For these reasons, exercise should be introduced gradually.

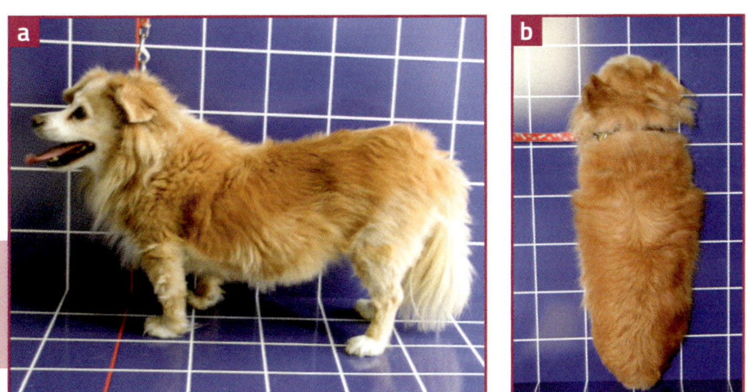

Figure 11. Overweight dog of advanced age. Appearance from dorsoventral view (b).

In addition to increasing caloric expenditure, sports training has other beneficial anti-obesity effects. The following are some of the advantages associated with exercise:[15–18]

- Muscle cells release proteins (myokines) with autocrine, paracrine, and endocrine activity. Myonectin, decorin, irisin, BDNF (brain-derived neurotrophic factor), and interleukins 1 and 10 are some of the myokines that affect muscle tissue growth, fatty acid oxidation and metabolism, short-term neuroendocrine control of energy intake, and synthesis of brown instead of white fat, as well as exerting anti-inflammatory effects.
- Angiogenesis and blood flow in adipose tissue are promoted, alleviating hypoxia.
- Local inflammation is diminished.
- In the endothelium, leukocyte adhesion and cytokine production are decreased.
- The immune system, which controls the number of proinflammatory cells and the production of cytokines, is activated.
- The secretion of growth hormone, which affects the relative proportions of lean and fatty tissue, is stimulated.
- Regulation of the endocannabinoid system, without the side effects of some drugs (e.g. rimonabant).

Further veterinary research will be required to corroborate these observations.

Finally, it has been shown that exercising with one's pet creates a more intense bond, contributes to a healthier life, and helps owners to better understand their pet's condition.[19–21] The type of physical activity in which the pet engages is largely determined by the owner's particular preferences. For example, some owners feel that it is not necessary to exercise cats, since they are sedentary animals and play alone (i.e. are self-sufficient). A minority of owners play with their cats, either for their own entertainment or to enhance their relationship with their pet. In the case of dogs, the type of sport will depend on breed and age (geriatric dogs are considered exempt), although daily activity, either alone or with other dogs in the park, is considered sufficient. The reasons for exercising with one's dog vary. Some owners may do so for their own sake. Others do so because it calms their pet, although in some cases exercise is limited owing to the risk of confrontations outside the home with other dogs or people.[4]

As animal health professionals, veterinary practitioners should inform and educate the public on these topics: changes in the dietary habits and physical activity of dogs and cats are necessary to prevent overweight.

PHARMACOLOGICAL TREATMENT OF OBESITY

The first treatment option for overweight is to change the patient's diet and eating habits. Exercise, as discussed above, contributes little to caloric expenditure. In the case of patients who do not reach their goals or whose behaviour is difficult to manage, medication may be an alternative option.

Drugs used for this purpose should have the following characteristics:
- Prescription medication (veterinary and/or human medicine).
- Safe, with few side effects and no toxic properties.
- Induce dose-dependent weight loss.
- Can be administered orally.
- Do not result in addiction or behavioural alterations.

Drugs can be classified according to their primary mechanism of action:
- Control of satiety and appetite: can act peripherally or centrally, as described below.
- Increase energy expenditure: not recommended owing to their adverse cardiovascular effects and their poor efficiency in inducing weight loss. Examples include caffeine, ephedrine, and L-thyroxine.
- Alterations in nutrient metabolism: already discussed in the section on dietary supplements in Chapter 5. Benefits are questionable.

Drugs with peripheral mode of action

Inhibitors of the microsomal triglyceride transfer protein

Dirlotapide[22] and mitratapide[23] are the only veterinary prescription drugs. They are indicated only for use in canids. Their mechanism of action is based on the sequestration of lipids in the endoplasmic reticulum of the enterocyte, hindering the synthesis and release of chylomicrons into the lymphatic system. They inhibit apolipoprotein B-48. This retention induces the release of peptide YY and glucagon-like peptide type 1 (GLP-1), which are responsible for decreasing food intake. Side effects include vomiting, diarrhoea, and steatorrhoea. These drugs can be administered at a fixed dose (mitratapide) or variable doses (dirlotapide) for a maximum period of 12 months (dirlotapide). It is recommended to accompany drug treatment with a prescription diet. Weight losses range from 8 % (mitratapide) to 18 % (dirlotapide). Currently these drugs are not authorised by the European Medicines Agency, nor are they available in the United States.

Pancreatic lipase inhibitors

Orlistatin is a pancreatic lipase inhibitor that reduces the absorption of dietary fat.[24] The observed weight loss is dose-dependent. Its effects are rapid (8 hours). Disadvantages associated with its use include a reduction in the absorption of apolar lipids (fat-soluble vitamins D and E, beta-carotene, and cholesterol), with no effect on polar lipids (fatty acids, bile acids, phospholipids, and vitamin A); steatorrhoea; flatulence; and the spontaneous elimination of diarrhoeal stools. Preclinical studies in dogs (<300 mg/kg/day) have demonstrated weight losses of approximately 4 % over a 1-year period. The manufacturer recommends coadministration of liposoluble multivitamin supplements. Orlistatin is not authorised for use in veterinary medicine.

GLP-1 agonists

Exenatide and liraglutide are synthetic GLP-1 agonists; liraglutide shares 97 % homology with the hormone. They are used to treat people with type 2 diabetes, and are administered parenterally twice daily or in a single dose. Interesting results have been obtained with liraglutide: significant weight reductions of 5 % and over 10 % have been reported after 56 weeks of treatment.[25] Both drugs have been experimentally tested for the treatment of feline diabetes in healthy and obese animals.[26,27] Cats treated for 7 days with subcutaneous liraglutide at 0.6 mg/cat showed a significant loss of appetite and a weight reduction of 9 %.[27] Side effects included emesis, diarrhoea, and anorexia. Further studies will be required to better evaluate its use in veterinary medicine, for which it is not currently authorised.

Central-acting drugs

Cannabinoid receptor blockers

Rimonabant is an antagonist of type 1 cannabinoid receptors. It decreases appetite (temporarily) as well as weight. The European Medicines Agency (EMA) and the United States Food and Drug Administration (FDA) have discontinued the commercialisation of rimonabant due to its serious neuropsychiatric effects in obese patients. Taranabant has not yet progressed beyond a phase III clinical trial. Oral administration of rimonabant in dogs at 1.25 mg/kg/day for 16 weeks resulted in significant decreases in food consumption (exclusively in the second week of treatment), subcutaneous fat (19.5 %), and body weight (2.5 %). At doses of 2.5 mg the following side effects are observed: anorexia, hypertension, and involuntary muscle contractions.[28] Its use in veterinary medicine is not authorised.

Serotonin agonists

Lorcaserin acts by activating serotonin receptors. In conjunction with diet and exercise, significant weight losses (5 % or more) have been reported in almost 50 % of treated individuals after 1 year of treatment. Adverse effects include cognitive and psychiatric disorders, priapism, and cardiopulmonary alterations.[29,30] No information on its use in veterinary medicine is available, nor is its use in veterinary medicine authorised.

Serotonin reuptake inhibitors

Sibutramine is an inhibitor of serotonin and noradrenaline reuptake. It acts by increasing satiety. Treatment of obese adults for 2 years has resulted in a weight loss of 10 %. Side effects are mainly cardiovascular and include hypertension and stroke. Sibutramine is not currently authorised for use in many countries, including EU member states and the United States.

In dogs, oral administration at 5 mg/kg 2 hours before offering the ration significantly increased gastric emptying and the volume of chyme in the duodenum, inhibited contraction of the small intestine, and resulted in feedback inhibition of stomach movements, inducing a sensation of intrameal satiety. Sibutramine acts both peripherally and centrally.[31] The authors provided no information on the extent of the weight loss achieved. Sibutramine is not authorised for use in veterinary medicine.

Fluoxetine is a selective sertotonin reuptake inhibitor that blocks the transport of serotonin from the synaptic cleft to the presynaptic terminal. It is used as an antidepressant and to treat obsessive-compulsive disorder. This drug works well as a short-term obesity treatment (less than 6 months). Treatment for longer periods is associated with a 50 % chance of a rebound effect. It is administered orally in dogs and cats at 1–2 mg/kg/day and 0.5–1 mg/kg/day, respectively. The varied associated side effects include behavioural changes (hyperactivity, irritability, and aggression).[32] In the United States it is marketed for veterinary use in patients with separation anxiety.

Noradrenergics

Phenylpropanolamine is an α-adrenergic drug. It suppresses appetite and promotes lipid catabolism. It is no longer used as an anorexigenic (an indication approved from 1975 to 1999) owing to the high risk of cerebral haemorrhage. In the EU it is prescribed at very low doses as an anti-flu drug (the toxic dose in adults is 100 mg). In veterinary medicine it is used for the control of urinary incontinence in female dogs (1–2 mg/kg every 8–12 hours) and occasionally in female cats.[32] Adverse clinical signs may be observed at doses of 1.9 mg/kg and higher, although the mean toxic dose is 29 mg/kg.[33] It is authorised for veterinary use in dogs only. No information is available on its use for the treatment of obesity in dogs or cats.

Combined treatment with opioid antagonists and dopamine reuptake inhibitors

The combination of naltrexone (a μ-opioid receptor antagonist) and bupropion (a weak inhibitor of dopamine reuptake that stimulates the secretion of proopiomelanocortin and β-endorphin) is one new treatment option for obesity. Both drugs have been shown to enhance each other's effects. Weight loss of 5–10 % is observed in treated patients over a period of 56 weeks.[34] There are no studies of their combined use in veterinary medicine. The two drugs have been used separately for the treatment of compulsive disorders in dogs and cats. The daily dose of naltrexone for dogs and cats is 2–5 mg/kg divided into 2 doses.[32] Bupropion at 1 mg/kg produces moderate depression, doses of 3–6 mg/kg cause pulmonary hypertension, and toxicity is observed at 10 mg/kg.[35] Neither of these two products are authorised for veterinary use.

SURGICAL TREATMENT OF OBESE PATIENTS

Bariatric surgery

Bariatric surgery constitutes an alternative to traditional treatments for obese people. Three main procedures are used: blocking, restricting, and mixed.[36] All are associated with potential complications,[37,38] including variable mortality ranging from 0.1 % (restrictive surgery) to 1.1 % (blocking surgery), dysphagia, reflux, cholelithiasis, pulmonary embolism, and sepsis. These techniques are not used in pets. Dogs and cats have been used as experimental models:[39] the electrical activity of the stomach has been studied in animals undergoing Roux-en-Y bypass (mixed), adjustable gastric banding (restricting), and biliopancreatic diversion (blocking).

Liposuction

The use of liposuction techniques is pets is recent, and little information is available in the literature.[40,41] In human medicine this technique (liposuction or liporeduction) has been widespread since the mid-1970s, owing to our obsession with body image. By contrast, in veterinary medicine it is used exclusively to eliminate large local fatty deposits. Large lipomas are usually found in obese, elderly animals and typically limit their movements or give rise to lesions caused by self-injury. We do not perform cosmetic procedures, but attempt to improve the patient's health.

Two surgical procedures are employed:

- Liposuction: a surgical aspirator and special cannulae are used to aspirate the fatty content. The advantages are that only a small incision is required and the procedure can be carried out with sedation and regional anaesthesia. The main drawbacks are marked bruising, ecchymosis, and seromas, as well as recurrence (1 in 4 animals), owing to the fact that the fibrous capsule is not removed. From our point of view, this is the technique of choice in animals with diffuse masses of 5–15 cm and owners who refuse to agree to surgery, although the owner should be advised that complete cure may not be achieved.
- Extraction: this is a surgical procedure performed under general anaesthesia. The advantage of this approach is that the lipoma, including its capsule, is completely eliminated, minimising the likelihood of recurrence.

Disadvantages include the need for a large incision, the risks associated with anaesthesia of senior patients, and the risk of seroma. It is the technique of choice for infiltrative nodules and for well-differentiated, small (<5 cm) or large (>15 cm) nodules (Figs. 12 and 13).

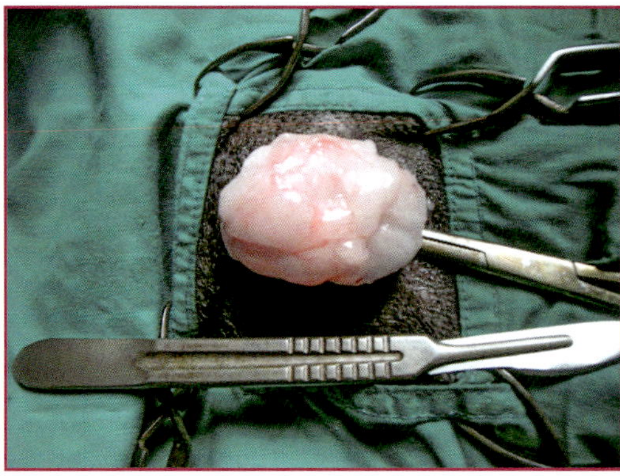

Figure 12. Nodule.

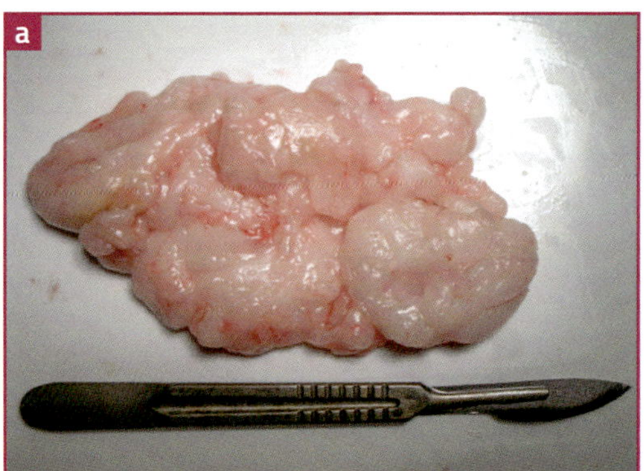

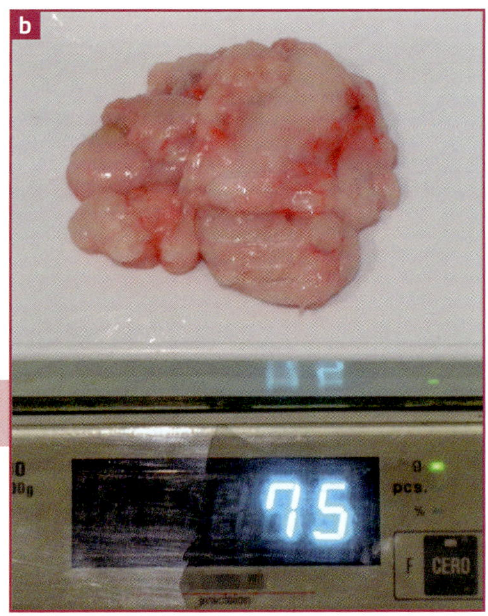

Figure 13. Extracted nodule (a) and weighing of same (b).

Case study 1

Figaro was a 12-year-old, 38.4-kg male Bobtail with a BCS of 7/9. He had a large diffuse nodule in the prescapular region and the right axilla that hindered movement. The owners were happy to accept the recommendations of the veterinary surgeon at all times. A preoperative study was carried out, and the patient was classified as ASA status II. Liposuction of the fat was performed using a surgical aspirator under sedation and local anaesthesia. The material removed equated to 500 ml and 440 g (1.15 % of the ideal weight). There was no recurrence over the following 15 months (the patient later died of cancer) (Fig. 14).

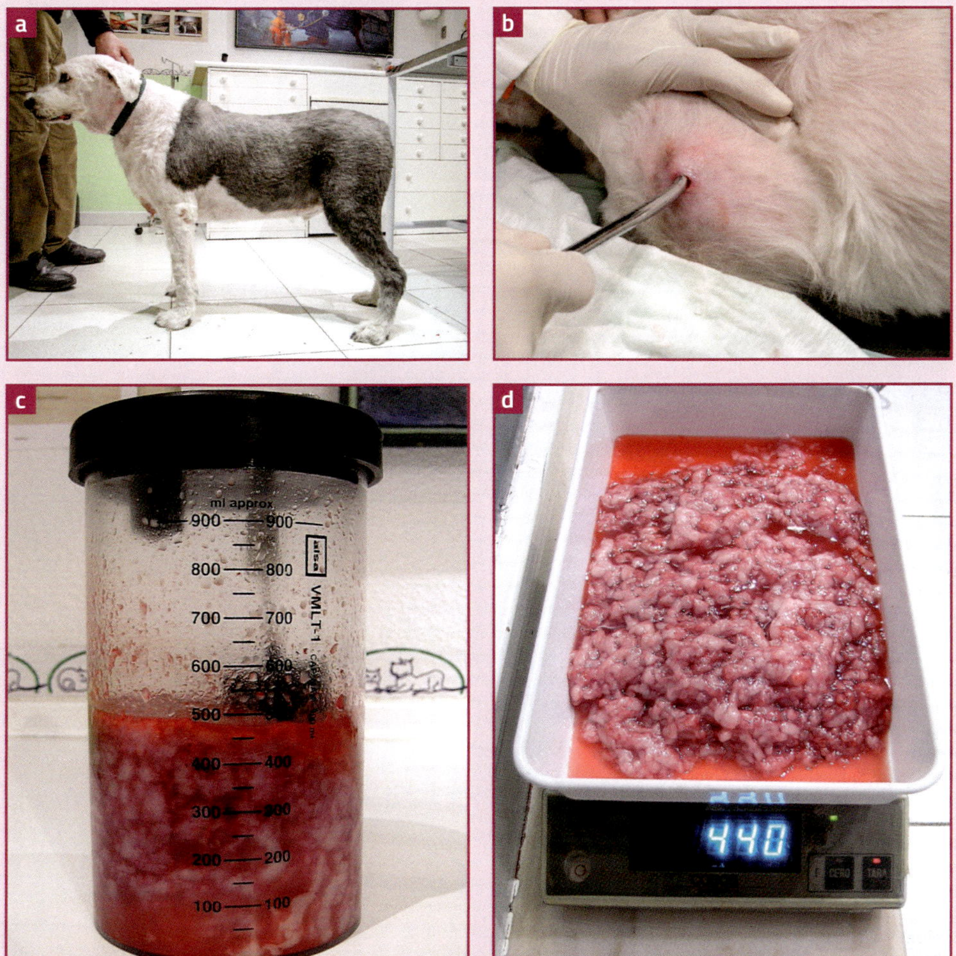

Figure 14. Patient (a) before undergoing the intervention for liposuction of the nodule contents (b). The fat removed corresponded to 500 ml (c) and 440 g (d).

8 Prevention of obesity

THE REBOUND OR YO-YO EFFECT

Once the patient's target weight has been reached, it is essential to maintain it over time. Reaching the target weight will also require readjustments throughout the course of the programme, and therefore the patient should be examined at regular intervals (every 30–50 days), depending on the owner's availability. Like in human medicine, in which 25–65 % of people who follow a weight-loss programme regain their lost weight, in veterinary medicine it is very difficult to maintain the target weight. Although data are scarce, a large number of animals appear to regain lost weight.

First, we will define what it means to maintain the target weight.

A weight-loss programme is considered successful when an individual intentionally loses at least 10 % of their initial weight and remains stable for at least 1 year.[1,2]

In our case we will substitute the individual with a pet. It is worth underscoring the use of the word "intentionally" (meaning as prescribed by a veterinary surgeon), and the specification of "a minimum of 1 year" (meaning more than just short-term weight loss). The best results are obtained when the target weight is maintained for more than 2 years. We can talk about complete success when the weight loss is maintained for the duration of the patient's life.

The yo-yo effect: underlying pathophysiology and factors involved

In studies carried out in rats, researchers found that the yo-yo effect is linked to the energetic difference created as a result of food restriction and reduced energy expenditure, resulting in compensatory hyperphagia when animals are provided with food, particularly fat-rich foods, as well as greater efficiency in its use (i.e. increased oxidation of carbohydrates and a suppression in fats). They found that the changes occurred within the first week, during which almost 40 % of the lost weight, which was mainly adipose tissue, was recovered, accompanied by a 30 % increase in the concentration of adipocytes per unit of adipose tissue (hyperplasia).[3–5] The likelihood of the rebound effect depends directly on the percentage of lost weight,[6] which is reduced with each successive cycle.[7] Studies have also described increases in the levels of lipoprotein-lipase and leptin, and of serum levels of triglycerides and cholesterol, resulting in a state of hyperlipogenesis.[8] These changes give rise to adipocyte enlargement and hyperplasia, lipid storage, increased leptin synthesis, possible alterations in the production of other cytokines, and changes in the hunger-satiety pattern that favour the development of disease.

In dogs the yo-yo effect is observed when fat-rich rewards are incorporated into the daily ration, possibly due to an increase in the palatability of the entire ration.[9,10,11]

Animals recovered weight more quickly (10 weeks versus 15 weeks), with higher daily gains (0.251 kg vs. 0.205 kg) and a higher percentage of body fat (41 % versus 40.2 %), despite the fact that their caloric intake was lower.[9]

In human medicine it has been shown that some hormonal changes may promote the rebound effect. Levels of amylin, leptin, ghrelin, peptide YY, GIP, and cholecystokinin are altered. Appetite changes have also been described. The concentrations of these hormones do not return to baseline levels (prior to the onset of overweight) and persist for 12 months.[12] In a person of optimal weight and in the absence of food or intense physical exercise, these changes would constitute an energy-saving/compensating mechanism, but this is not the case in an environment in which food is abundant and physical activity is minimal.

Although the vast majority of the factors involved in the rebound effect in humans are behavioural in nature, some are associated with nutrition:

- High levels of dietary protein appear to favour weight maintenance.[13] However, not all studies have produced concordant results.
- Certain micronutrients influence the expression of some genes associated with adipose tissue stress and inflammation. Ingestion of micronutrients with anti-inflammatory effects is negatively correlated with the rebound effect. Effects have been demonstrated for some micronutrients, either alone or in combination with exercise: magnesium (reduces oxidative stress), folic acid (reduces inflammatory signals in obese patients), and riboflavin or vitamin B_2 (reduces levels of some proinflammatory factors such as TNF-α and IL-6). By contrast, positive correlations have been observed for nutrients with proinflammatory effects, such as carbohydrates, total fat, saturated fats, cholesterol, and energy (from the point of view of nutrition, energy is considered a nutrient).[14]
- Certain flavonoids synthesised by the digestive microbiota, known as postbiotics (apigenin and naringenin), promote increased energy expenditure through increased expression of uncoupling protein 1 (UCP-1). Studying their value in the prevention of obesity and the yo-yo effect constitutes a new avenue of research.[15]

Preventive strategies

Strategies used in human medicine[16–25] should be used as reference points in veterinary medicine, and adapted to canine and feline patients (Fig. 1):

- **Control of daily caloric intake and food characteristics.** The daily maintenance energy requirements of dogs and cats have been well defined for many years. In both species, equations have been proposed to calculate requirements, taking multiple factors into account.[11,26–28] Given the current lifestyle of our patients, these estimates need to be redefined. When dealing with animals that engage in little activity and are confined to the home, calculation of the daily requirements of dogs and cats can be simplified by taking 75–80 % of the result of Equations 3 and 4 in Chapter 6 proposed by the NRC (2006). Once again, it will be necessary to readjust the requirements to avoid changes in body weight over time, as discussed in Chapter 6 (Fig. 2). There are no defined standards regarding food characteristics. We can continue with the usual maintenance formula or with one that has a lower energy density (e.g. labelled "low in calories" or "for weight control"). It is important to make the transition gradually to avoid possible digestive disorders or anxiety related to the novelty of the ration.

- **Increase in physical activity.** This has little impact on energetic balance but does help owners and their pets to bond. As revealed by epidemiological studies of obesity in pets, owners may find it difficult to ensure that their pet exercises daily. It is not uncommon to see young owners sitting on a bench using their cell phone or eating a snack with their dog next to them, sharing the snack. By contrast, it is very common to see older people, often retirees, regularly walking their dogs.
- **Distribute the food in three portions**, with the largest offered in the morning (e.g. using a 60:20:20 ratio). Currently, the typical regimen is one portion in the morning and another in the evening.
- **Periodic monitoring of weight and body condition.** This can be done at home (using a bathroom scales for medium-sized cats and dogs) or at the veterinary centre. Visits scheduled as part of the patient's health programme (e.g. vaccinations, deworming) provide a good opportunity to perform these measurements.
- **Clinical follow-up of patients who have completed the treatment programme.** The work of veterinary assistants is essential when it comes to coordinating these examinations, either by phone, online, or using mobile applications (apps). Veterinary surgeons either supervise or directly participate in this examination (it is important that the owner and their pet receive personalised attention). While many owners are uncomfortable with these processes, as also occurs in human medicine, their efficacy in treating the disease in the long term is well demonstrated.
- **Self-control of the owner:** the owner must be disciplined in implementing the recommended feeding habits throughout the dietetic programme (Fig. 3).
- **Record information** on diet, weight, and physical activity by systematically collecting data (type of diet, quantity offered, extra food, exercise, etc.) in a diary or an app for subsequent discussion and analysis with the clinical team.
- **Do not succumb to peer pressure.** It is common that when out for a walk other pet owners will question the optimal weight proposed for the pet. The efforts made to treat the patient must not be undermined by the opinions of nonprofessionals.
- **Attend meetings with other owners** whose pets have successfully completed a weight-loss programme in order to hear the experiences of the other owners. While we have found no reports of the use of this approach in veterinary medicine, it appears to provide good results in human medicine.

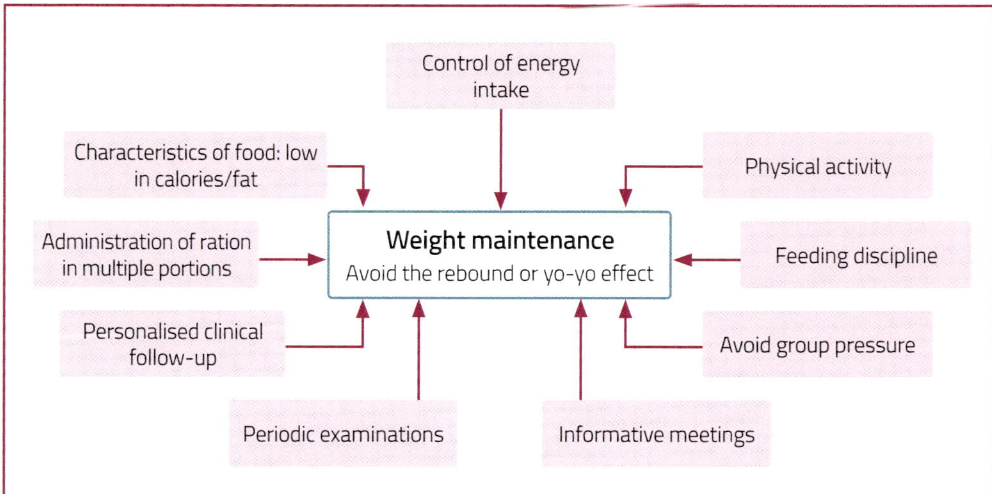

Figure 1. Prevention strategies.

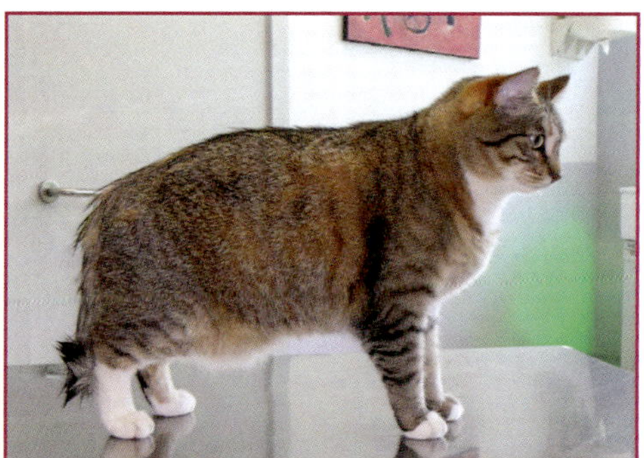

Figure 2. This patient currently weighs 7.2 kg, has a BCS of 7/9, and has just started a weight-loss programme. After 12–17 weeks, at the end of the programme, the patient's daily requirements are calculated at 265.74 kcal ME: [80 %$(100 \times 6^{0.67})$].

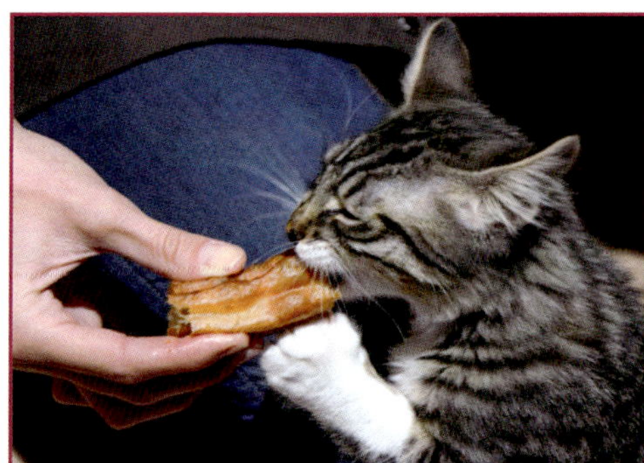

Figure 3. The owner must be alert, and should not offer their pet inappropriate foods.

MONITORING DURING DIFFERENT STAGES

Monitoring during growth

When dealing with developing animals, it is important to note their position on the growth curve. To this end, it is necessary to know the age of the pet, or at least their dental age, the corresponding growth curve, and the point at which growth ends. Based on prediction equations and estimations of the mean weight gain, some curves/tables have been prepared to allow us to predict the weight of a puppy at each stage of life, and thereby determine their specific requirements.[11,29]

In cats, the mean weight gain is 100 g per week during the first 6 months of life. Sex-related differences in growth are very evident after 4 weeks of age: females grow more slowly and have a lower adult weight than males. Growth slows from this point on; males gain a mean of 20 g/day, while females gain approximately half this amount. Growth is completed (closure of growth plates) at 10 months of age (Fig. 4).

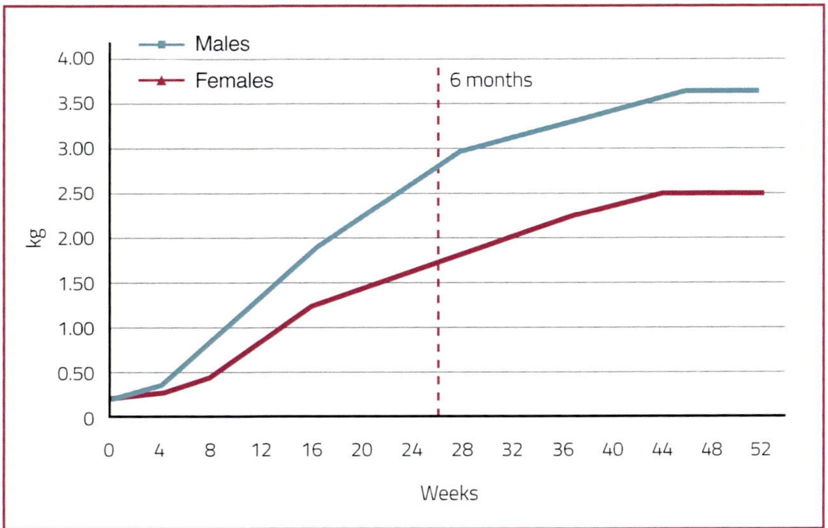

Figure 4. Growth curves for cats according to sex.

All dog breeds reach approximately 50 % of their adult weight between 4 and 5 months of age. From this point until the end of the growth process (adulthood) there are marked differences between breeds. Large and giant breeds take twice as long to reach maturity (Fig. 5). Small and medium breeds reach 80 % of their adult weight at 9–10 months and complete growth at 12 months, while large/giant breeds reach 80 % of their adult weight at 11–15 months and complete growth by 18–24 months (Fig. 6). Table 1 provides an estimate of body weight at each stage.

Calculation of the daily requirements of dogs and cats is summarised in Table 2.

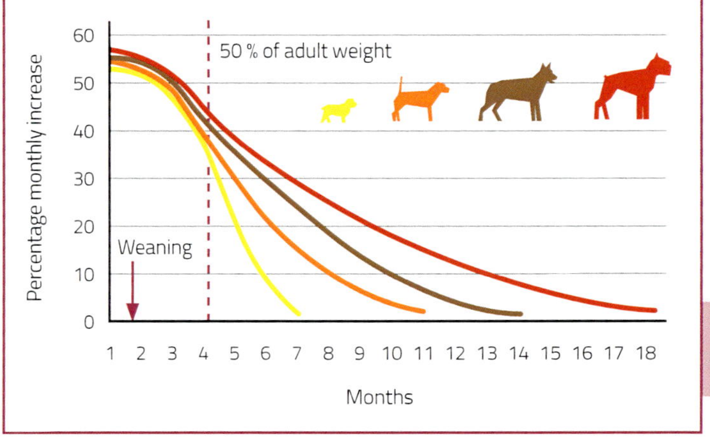

Figure 5. Mean weight gain curves for dogs, according to size.

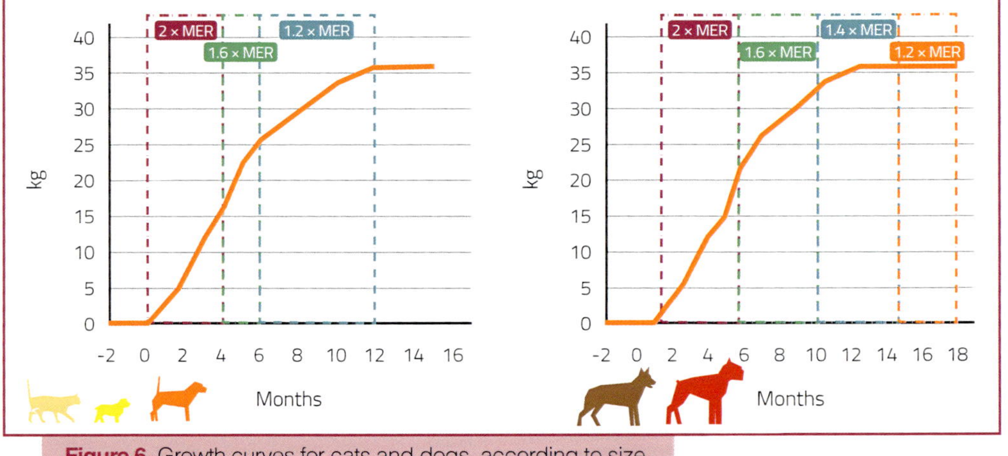

Figure 6. Growth curves for cats and dogs, according to size.

Weeks of age	Mean daily gain or percentage of adult weight in dogs
1	8 % current weight
2	6 % current weight
3	4 % current weight
4	3.5 % current weight
4–8	3 g/kg adult weight
>8	2–4 g/kg adult weight
16	50 % adult weight (dogs <25 kg)
20	50 % adult weight (dogs >25 kg)
32	65 % adult weight
>40	80 % adult weight
40–60	100 % adult weight (depending on breed)
48–96	Complete development (depending on breed)

Table 1. Estimation of dog's weight according to age.

Table 2. Energy requirements during growth.

<table>
<tr><th rowspan="2">Age</th><th colspan="7">ER_{growth} = × MER</th></tr>
<tr><th>Birth–week 2</th><th>Week 2–weaning</th><th>Weaning–4 months</th><th>4–6 months</th><th>6–10 months</th><th colspan="2">10–12 months</th></tr>
<tr><td>Small and medium dogs</td><td rowspan="3">0.55</td><td>1.9</td><td>2</td><td>1.6</td><td>1.2</td><td colspan="2">1</td></tr>
<tr><td rowspan="2">Large and giant dogs</td><td rowspan="2">2.3</td><td>Weaning–4 months</td><td>4–8 months</td><td>9–12 months</td><td>12–18 months</td><td>18–24 months</td></tr>
<tr><td>2</td><td>1.6</td><td>1.4</td><td>1.2</td><td>1</td></tr>
<tr><td rowspan="2">Cats</td><td>Birth–week 2</td><td>Week 2–weaning</td><td>Weaning-5 months</td><td>5–6 months</td><td>7–8.5 months</td><td>9–11 months</td><td>12 months</td></tr>
<tr><td>1.6</td><td>2–2.5</td><td>2.5</td><td>1.7</td><td>1.4</td><td>1.2</td><td>1</td></tr>
</table>

Example

A 5-month-old puppy of average size for his breed weighs 8 kg or approximately 80 % of his adult weight (14 kg). His daily requirements can be calculated using the following equation:

$ER_{growth} = MER_{dogs}{}^{*} \times 3.2 \times [e^{(-0.87p)} - 0.1]$

Or: $ER_{growth} = 1.6 \times MER_{dogs}{}^{*}$

The daily requirement will be 1,005 kcal ME/day. Next, the daily ration will have to be adjusted to the energy content of the selected food.

* Equation 3, Chapter 6.

We find ourselves dealing with a new field within veterinary medicine: paediatrics. If monthly examinations are performed throughout the first year of a child's life, then why not do the same in veterinary medicine?

Several processes occur at this stage of our patients' lives that are closely related to the onset of overweight. Learning, hierarchy, social behaviour, and training are sometimes reinforced using food as a reward, resulting in an increase in the number of calories consumed and stimulation of the neural areas that link food with pleasure.

Appropriate evolution of size and weight in dogs and cats is the first preventive factor for overweight.

Monitoring in adult patients

We have already discussed the factors that predispose animals to overweight and the yo-yo effect. Correct control of these factors by the veterinary team and education of the owners are only preventive measures (Fig. 7).

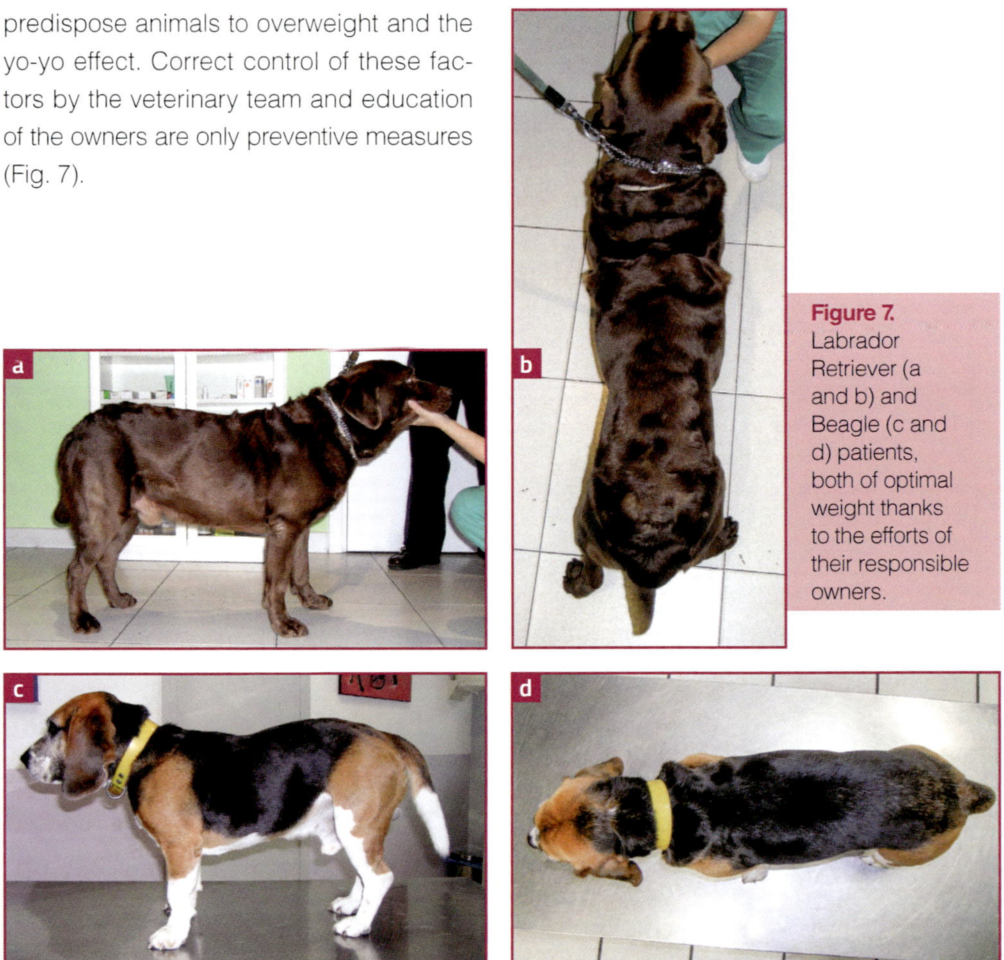

Figure 7. Labrador Retriever (a and b) and Beagle (c and d) patients, both of optimal weight thanks to the efforts of their responsible owners.

Neutered animals

Approximately 30–40 % of dogs and over 60 % of cats are neutered. The age at which animals are neutered varies, and depends on the species: cats are neutered at younger ages, while in dogs there is no clearly defined moment at which this procedure should be performed. The changes associated with gonadectomy are discussed in Chapter 1, and should be taken into account when making decisions once the animal has been neutered (Fig. 8).

The requirements of these patients will be conditioned by the age at which they are neutered and their subsequent management in adulthood. Taking into account the animal's development, which, as mentioned previously, affects the adipose tissue, it will also be necessary to modify requirements during the growth stage and to readjust them in adulthood.

Below, we will review these concepts in the context of the theoretical calculation of the energetic requirements of a cat[11,29] (a species in which neutering is very common).

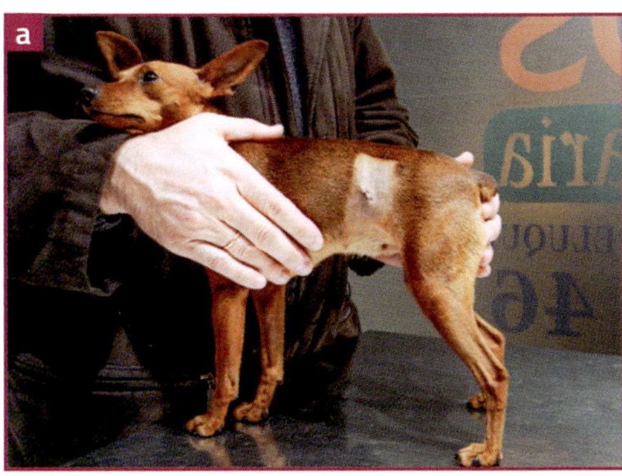

Figure 8. Patient that has undergone ovariohysterectomy (a). Images taken during surgery (b and c).

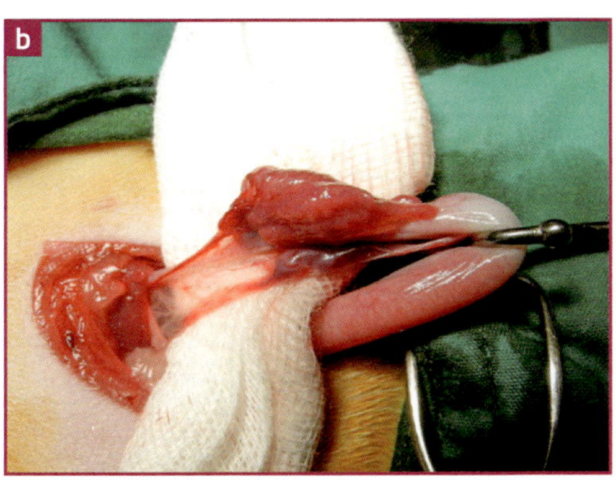

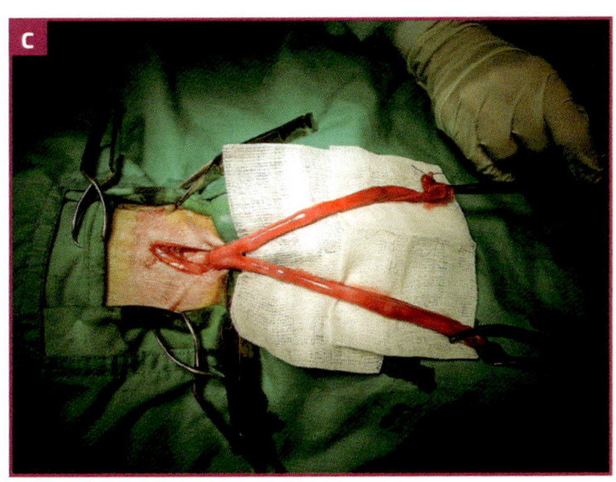

Example

Melendis, adopted at 2 months, was neutered at 7 months of age with a body weight (BW) of 4 kg (80 % of adult weight) (Fig. 9).

The calculations are as follows:

MER_{cat} (kcal ME/day) * = $100 \times BW^{0.67}$

$MER_{growth\ cat}$ (kcal ME/day)$_{phase\ I}$ = $1.4 \times [100 \times 4^{0.67}]$

MER (kcal ME/day)$_{phase\ I}$ = 354 kcal ME/day, until the moment of surgery.

$MER_{growth\ cat}$ (kcal ME/day)$_{phase\ II}$ = $1.2 \times [100 \times 4.6^{0.67}] \times 80$ %

MER (kcal ME/day)$_{phase\ II}$ = 267 kcal ME/day, up to 12 months.

Energy of specific food = 346 kcal ME/100 g

Daily amount of food in phase I = 354 kcal/day: 3.46 kcal/g = 102 g/day

Daily amount of food in phase II = 267 kcal/day: 3.46 kcal/g = 77 g/day

After 12 months, the daily requirements were 80 % of those calculated for maintenance, or 235 kcal ME/day, with a ration of 68 g/day (Fig. 10).

* Equation 4, Chapter 6.

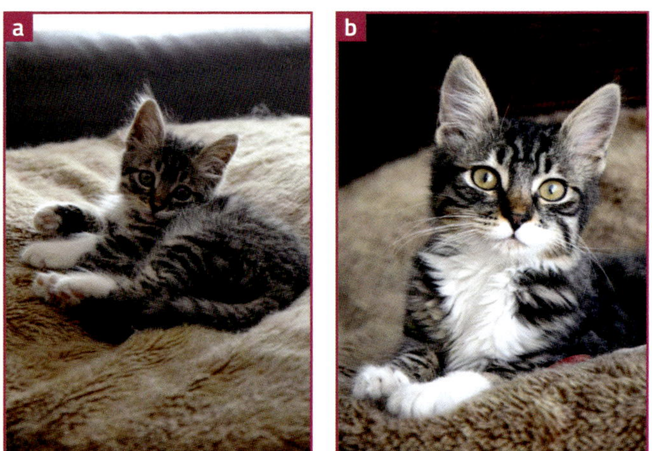

Figure 9. *Melendis* at 2 months (a) and 5 months (b) of age.

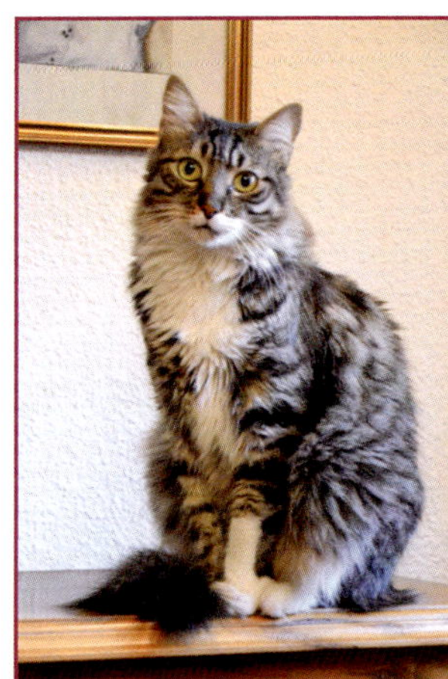

Figure 10. *Melendis* at 2 years of age.

References

Chapter 1. General aspects of obesity

1. Kirk, C. In: Gorman J. Survival of the fattest: How pets got so big. *New York Times*, 2003 September 16.
2. Kealy RD, Lawler DF, Ballam JM, et al. Effects of diet restriction on life span and age-related changes in dogs. *J Am Vet Med Assoc*, 2002; 220(9):1315–1320.
3. Yam PS, Butowski CF, Chitty JL, et al. Impact of canine overweight and obesity on health-related quality of life. *Prev Vet Med*, 2016 May 1; 127:64–69.
4. Lake A, Townshend T. Obesogenic environments: exploring the built and food environments. *J R Soc Promot Health*, 2006 Nov; 126(6):262–267.
5. Martin AA, Davidson TL. Human cognitive function and the obesogenic environment. *Physiol Behav*, 2014 Sep; 136:185–193.
6. Mackenbach JD, Rutter H, Compernolle S, et al. Obesogenic environments: a systematic review of the association between the physical environment and adult weight status, the SPOTLIGHT project. *BMC Public Health*, 2014 Mar 6; 14:233.
7. Domecq JP, Prutsky G, Leppin A, et al. Clinical review: Drugs commonly associated with weight change: a systematic review and meta-analysis. *J Clin Endocrinol Metab*, 2015 Feb; 100(2):363–370.
8. Corbee RJ. Obesity in show cats. *J Anim Physiol Anim Nutr (Berl)*, 2014; 98(6):1075–1080.
9. Corbee RJ. Obesity in show dogs. *J Anim Physiol Anim Nutr (Berl)*, 2013; 97(5): 904–910.
10. Courcier EA, Mellor DJ, Pendlebury E, et al. An investigation into the epidemiology of feline obesity in Great Britain: results of a cross-sectional study of 47 companion animal practises. *Vet Rec*, 2012 Dec 1; 171(22):560.
11. Courcier EA, Thomson RM, Mellor DJ, Yam PS. An epidemiological study of environmental factors associated with canine obesity. *J Small Anim Pract*, 2010; 51(7):362–367.
12. Edney AT, Smith PM. Study of obesity in dogs visiting veterinary practices in the United Kingdom. *Vet Rec*, 1986 Apr 5; 118(14):391–396.
13. Lund EM, Armstrong PJ, Kirk CA, Klausner JS. Prevalence and risk factors for obesity in adult dogs from private US veterinary practices. *Int J Appl Res Vet Med*, 2006; 4:177–186.
14. Lund EM, Armstrong PJ, Kirk CA, Klausner JS. Prevalence and risk factors for obesity in adult cats from private US veterinary practices. *Int J Appl Res Vet Med*, 2005; 3:88–96.
15. Mao J, Xia Z, Chen J, Yu J. Prevalence and risk factors for canine obesity surveyed in veterinary practices in Beijing, China. *Prev Vet Med*, 2013 Nov 1; 112(3-4):438–442.
16. McGreevy PD, Thomson PC, Pride C, et al. Prevalence of obesity in dogs examined by Australian veterinary practices and the risk factors involved. *Vet Rec*, 2005; 156(22):695–702.
17. Mussa PP, Prola L, Meineri G. Obesity in dog: a survey results in Italy. *Proceedings of the 10th Congress of the European Society of Veterinary and Comparative Nutrition*. Nantes, France, 2006.
18. Sandøe P, Palmer C, Corr S, Astrup A, Bjørnvad CR. Canine and feline obesity: a One Health perspective. *Vet Rec*, 2014; 175(24):610–616.

19. Tarkosova D, Story MM, Rand JS, Svoboda M. Feline obesity-prevalence, risk factors, pathogenesis, associated conditions and assessment: a review. *Vet Med (Praha)*, 2016; 61(6):295–307.

20. Usui S, Yasuda H, Koketsu Y. Characteristics of obese or overweight dogs visiting private Japanese veterinary clinics. *Asian Pac J Trop Biomed*, 2016 April; 6(4):338–343.

21. Weeth LP, Fascetti AJ, Kass PH, et al. Prevalence of obese dogs in a population of dogs with cancer. *Am J Vet Res*, 2007; 68(4):389–398.

22. Laflamme DP, Abood SK, Fascetti AJ, et al. Pet feeding practices of dog and cat owners in the United States and Australia. *J Am Vet Med Assoc*, 2008 Mar 1; 232(5):687–694.

23. Kienzle E, Bergler R, Mandernach A. A comparison of the feeding behavior and the human-animal relationship in owners of normal and obese dogs. *J Nutr*, 1998; 128:2779S–2782S.

24. Cavalieri-Carciofi A, Nogueira-Venturelli K, Souza-Vasconcellos R, et al. A weight loss protocol and owners participation in the treatment of canine obesity. *Cienc Rural*, Santa Maria, 2005 Nov/Dec; 35(6):1331–1338.

25. Öhlund M, Palmgren M, Holst BS. Overweight in adult cats: a cross-sectional study. *Acta Vet Scand*, 2018; 60(1):5.

26. Raffan E, Dennis RJ, O'Donovan CJ, et al. A deletion in the canine POMC gene is associated with weight and appetite in obesity-prone Labrador Retriever dogs. *Cell Metab*, 2016 May 10; 23(5):893–900.

27. Häring T, Wichert B, Dolf G, Haase B. Segregation analysis of overweight body condition in an experimental cat population. *J Hered*, 2011; 102(Suppl 1):S28–S31.

28. Ishioka K, Hosoya K, Kitagawa H, et al. Plasma leptin concentration in dogs: effects of body condition score, age, gender and breeds. *Res Vet Sci*, 2007; 82(1):11–15.

29. Jeusette I, Greco D, Aquino F, et al. Effect of breed on body composition and comparison between various methods to estimate body composition in dogs. *Res Vet Sci*, 2010 Apr; 88(2):227–232.

30. Park HJ, Lee SE, Oh JH, et al. Leptin, adiponectin and serotonin levels in lean and obese dogs. *BMC Vet Res*, 2014; 10:113.

31. Plassais J, Rimbault M, Williams FJ, et al. Analysis of large versus small dogs reveals three genes on the canine X chromosome associated with body weight, muscling and back fat thickness. *PLoS Genet*, 2017 Mar 3; 13(3):e1006661.

32. Mendez IA, Ostlund SB, Maidment NT, Murphy NP. Involvement of endogenous enkephalins and β-endorphin in feeding and diet-induced obesity. *Neuropsychopharmacology*, 2015; 40(9):2103–2112.

33. Colliard L, Paragon BM, Lemuet B, et al. Prevalence and risk factors of obesity in an urban population of healthy cats. *J Feline Med Surg*, 2009 Feb; 11(2):135–140.

34. Spain CV, Scarlett JM, Houpt KA. Long-term risks and benefits of early-age gonadectomy in cats. *J Am Vet Med Assoc*, 2004 Feb 1; 224(3):372–379.

35. Spain CV, Scarlett JM, Houpt KA. Long-term risks and benefits of early-age gonadectomy in dogs. *J Am Vet Med Assoc*, 2004 Feb 1; 224 (3):380–387.

36. Kanchuk ML, Backus RC, Calvert CC, et al. Neutering induces changes in food intake, body weight, plasma insulin and leptin concentrations in normal and lipoprotein lipase-deficient male cats. *J Nutr*, 2002; 132:1730S–1732S.

37. Backus RC, Kanchuk ML, Rogers QR. Elevation of plasma cholecystokinin concentration following a meal is increased by gonadectomy in male cats. J *Anim Physiol Anim Nutr (Berl)*, 2006 Apr; 90(3–4):152–158.

38. Kanchuk ML, Backus RC, Calvert CC, et al. Weight gain in gonadectomized normal and lipoprotein lipase-deficient male domestic cats results from increased food intake and not decreased energy expenditure. *J Nutr*, 2003; 133(6):1866–1874.

39. Martin LJ, Siliart B, Dumon HJ, Nguyen P. Spontaneous hormonal variations in male cats following gonadectomy. *J Feline Med Surg*, 2006; 8(5):309-314.

40. Jeusette I, Detilleux J, Cuvelier C, et al. Ad libitum feeding following ovariectomy in female Beagle dogs: effect on maintenance energy requirements and on blood metabolites. *J Anim Phisiol Anim Nutr (Berl)*, 2004 Apr; 88(3–4):117–121.
41. Belsito KR, Vester BM, Keel T, et al. Impact of ovariohysterectomy and food intake on body composition, physical activity, and adipose gene expression in cats. *J Anim Sci*, 2009; 87(2):594–602.
42. Nguyen PG, Dumon HJ, Siliart BS, et al. Effects of dietary fat and energy on body weight and composition after gonadectomy in cats. *Am J Vet Res*, 2004 Dec; 65(12):1708–1713.
43. Cooke PS, Naaz A. Role of estrogens in adipocyte development and function. *Exp Biol Med (Maywood)*, 2004 Dec; 229(11):1127–1135.
44. Le Roux PH. Thyroid status, oestradiol level, work performance and body mass of ovariectomised bitches and bitches bearing ovarian autotransplants in the stomach wall. *J S Afr Vet Assoc*, 1983; 54(2):115–117.
45. Kopelman PG. Physiopathology of prolactin secretion in obesity. *Int J Obes Retal Metab Disord*, 2000; 24(Suppl 2):S104–S108.
46. Louveau I, Gondret F. Regulation of development and metabolism of adipose tissue by growth hormone and the insulin-like growth factor system. *Domest Anim Endocrinol*, 2004; 27(3):241–255.
47. Martin LJ, Siliart B, Dumon HJ, Nguyen PG. Hormonal disturbances associated with obesity in dogs. *J Anim Physiol Anim Nutr (Berl)*, 2006 Oct; 90(9–10):355–360.
48. Bjornvad CR, Rand JS, Tan HY, et al. Obesity and sex influence insulin resistance and total and multimer adiponectin levels in adult neutered domestic shorthair client-owned cats. *Domest Anim Endocrinol*, 2014 Apr;47:55–64.
49. World Health Organization. *WHO Obesity and overweight. Global Health Observatory data.* World health statistics, 2018 Feb.
50. Kienzle E, Bergler R. Human-animal relationship of owners of normal and overweight cats. *J Nutr*, 2006 Jul; 136(7 Suppl):1947S–1950S.
51. Colliard L, Ancel J, Benet JJ, et al. Risk factors for obesity in dogs in France. *J Nutr*, 2006 Jul; 136(7 Suppl):1951S–1954S.
52. Parry LL, Netuveli G, Parry J, Saxena S. A systematic review of parental perception of overweight status in children. *J Ambul Care Manage*, 2008 Jul–Sep; 31(3):253–268.
53. White GA, Hobson-West P, Cobb K, et al. Canine obesity: is there a difference between veterinarian and owner perception? *J Small Anim Pract*, 2011; 52(12):622–626.
54. Akinrinmade F, Akinrinde AS. Nutritional composition and label evaluation of some commercial dry dog foods in Ibadan, Nigeria. *Afr J Biomed Res*, 2011 May; 14:157–160.
55. Davies M, Alborough R, Jones L, et al. Mineral analysis of complete dog and cat foods in the UK and compliance with European guidelines. *Sci Rep*, 2017; 7(1):17107.
56. Handl S, Danninger-Dobrovits C, Iben C. Do feeding instructions on commercial dog foods promote obesity? In: Szymeczko R, Iben C, Burlikowska K, et al. (eds.). *Proceedings of the 16th Congress of the European Society of Veterinary and Comparative Nutrition*. Bydgoszcz (Poland): Multikop Sp. Z, 2012. p. 3.
57. Hill RC, Choate CJ, Scott KC, Molenberghs G. Comparison of the guaranteed analysis with the measured nutrient composition of commercial pet foods. *J Am Vet Med Assoc*, 2009 Feb 1; 234(3):347–351.
58. Rolinec M, Biro D, Gálik B, et al. The nutritive value of selected commercial dry dog foods. *Acta fytotechn zootechn*, 2016; 19(1):25–28.
59. Sallander M, Hedhammar A, Rundgren M, Lindberg JE. *A study on the nutrient and energy content of commercial dog feeds*; 2001. https://pub.epsilon.slu.se/1501/6/MarSalFINAL5.pdf
60. Rowe E, Browne W, Casey R, et al. Risk factors identified for owner-reported feline obesity at around one year of age: Dry diet and indoor lifestyle. *Prev Vet Med*, 2015 Oct 1; 121(3–4):273–281.
61. Rowe EC, Browne WJ, Casey RA, et al. Early-life risk factors identified for owner-reported feline overweight and obesity at around two years of age. *Prev Vet Med*, 2017 Aug 1; 143:39–48.

62. Zoran DL. The carnivore connection to nutrition in cats. *J Am Vet Med Assoc*, 2002 Dec 1; 221(11):1559–1567.
63. Holmes KL, Morris PJ, Abdulla Z, et al. Risk factors associated with excess body weight in dogs in the UK. *J Anim Physiol Anim Nutr*, 2007 April; 91(3–4):166–167.
64. Nijland ML, Stam F, Seidell JC. Overweight in dogs, but not in cats, is related to overweight in their owners. *Public Health Nutr*, 2010 Jan; 13(1):102–106.
65. Russell K, Sabin R, Holt S, et al. Influence of feeding regimen on body condition in the cat. *J Small Anim Pract*, 2000 Jan; 41(1):12–17.
66. Bland IM, Guthrie-Jones A, Taylor RD, Hill J. Dog obesity: owner attitudes and behaviour. *Prev Vet Med*, 2009; 92(4):333–340.
67. Ministerio de Sanidad, Servicios Sociales e Igualdad. *Estrategia NAOS*. http://www.aecosan.msssi.gob.es/AECOSAN/web/nutricion/seccion/estrategia_naos.htm
68. Sánchez-Romero M. El consumo de alimento como estrategia social: recetas para la construcción de la memoria y la creación de identidades. *Cuadernos de prehistoria y arqueología de la Universidad de Granada*, 2008; 18:17–39. ISSN 0211-3228.
69. White GA, Ward L, Pink C, et al. "Who's been a good dog?" – owner perceptions and motivations for treat giving. *Prev Vet Med*, 2016; 132:14–19.
70. Nightingale CE, Margarson MP, Shearer E, et al. Peri-operative management of the obese surgical patient 2015: Association of Anaesthetists of Great Britain and Ireland Society for Obesity and Bariatric Anaesthesia. *Anaesthesia*, 2015 Jul; 70(7):859–876.
71. Van Goethem BE, Rosenveldt KW, Kirpensteijn J. Monopolar versus bipolar electrocoagulation in canine laparoscopic ovariectomy: a nonrandomized, prospective, clinical trial. *Vet Surg*, 2003 Sep–Oct; 32(5):464–470.
72. Forse RA, Karam B, MacLean LD, Christou NV. Antibiotic prophylaxis for surgery in morbidly obese patients. *Surgery*, 1989 Oct; 106(4):750–756; discussion 756–757.
73. Guo S, Dipietro LA. Factors affecting wound healing. *J Dent Res*, 2010 Mar; 89(3):219–229.
74. Winfield RD, Reese S, Bochicchio K, et al. Obesity and the risk for surgical site infection in abdominal surgery. *Am Surg*, 2016 Apr; 82(4):331–336.
75. Pierpont YN, Dinh TP, Salas RE, et al. Obesity and surgical wound healing: a current review. *ISRN Obes*, 2014; 2014:638936.
76. Pai MP. Drug dosing based on weight and body surface area: mathematical assumptions and limitations in obese adults. *Pharmacotherapy*, 2012 Sep; 32(9):856–868.
77. Ingrande J, Lemmens HJ. Dose adjustment of anaesthetics in the morbidly obese. *Br J Anaesth*, 2010 Dec; 105(Suppl 1):i16–23.
78. Parameswaran K, Todd DC, Soth M. Altered respiratory physiology in obesity. *Can Respir J*, 2006 May-Jun; 13(4):203–210.
79. Manens J, Bolognin M, Bernaerts F, et al. Effects of obesity on lung function and airway reactivity in healthy dogs. *Vet J*, 2012; 193(1):217–221.
80. Bach JF, Rozanski EA, Bedenice D, et al. Association of expiratory airway dysfunction with marked obesity in healthy adult dogs. *Am J Vet Res*, 2007; 68(6):670–675.
81. Boutheguard JC, Kelly M, Clety N, et al. Effects of weight loss on heart rate normalization and increase in spontaneous activity in moderately exercised overweight dogs. *Int J Appl Res Vet Med*, 2009; 7(4):153–164.
82. López-Jiménez F, Cortés-Bergoderi M. Obesidad y corazón. *Rev Esp Cardiol*, 2011; 64(02):140–149.
83. Thengchaisri N, Theerapun W, Kaewmokul S, Sastravaha A. Abdominal obesity is associated with heart disease in dogs. *BMC Vet Res*, 2014; 10:131.
84. Tropf M, Nelson OL, Lee PM, Weng HY. Cardiac and metabolic variables in obese dogs. *J Vet Intern Med*, 2017 Jul–Aug; 31(4):1000–1007.
85. Tvarijonaviciute A, Ceron JJ, Holden SL, et al. Obesity-related metabolic dysfunction in dogs: a comparison with human metabolic syndrome. *BMC Vet Res*, 2012; 8:147.
86. Truett AA, Borne AT, Poincot MA, West DB. Autonomic control of blood pressure and heart rate in obese hypertensive dogs. *Am J Physiol*, 1996; 270(3):R541–549.

87. Bille C, Auvigne V, Libermann S, et al. Risk of anaesthetic mortality in dogs and cats: an observational cohort study of 3546 cases. *Vet Anaesth Analg*, 2012 Jan; 39(1):59–68.
88. Brodbelt D. Perioperative mortality in small animal anaesthesia. *Vet J*, 2009 Nov; 182(2):152–161.
89. Brodbelt DC, Blissitt KJ, Hammond RA, et al. The risk of death: the confidential enquiry into perioperative small animal fatalities. *Vet Anaesth Analg*, 2008 Sep; 35(5):365–373.
90. Patel AM. Appropriate consent and referral for general anaesthesia – a survey in the Paediatric Day Care Unit, Barnsley DGH NHS Trust, South Yorkshire. *Br Dent J*, 2004 Mar 13; 196(5):275–277.

Chapter 2. Adipose tissue

1. Langin D, Frühbeck G, Frayn KN. Adipose tissue: development, anatomy and functions. In: *Obesity: science to practice*. Oxford, UK: Wiley-Blackwell, J. Wiley & sons, Ltd, 2009; Chapter 4, pp. 79–108.
2. Rasouli N, Kern PA. Adipocytokines and the metabolic complications of obesity. *J Clin Endocrinol Metab*, 2008 Nov; 93(11 Suppl 1):S64–S73.
3. Tang W, Zeve D, Suh JM, et al. White fat progenitor cells reside in the adipose vasculature. *Science*, 2008; 322(5901):583–586.
4. Virtanen KA, Lidell ME, Orava J, et al. Functional brown adipose tissue in healthy adults. *N Engl J Med*, 2009; 360:1518–1525.
5. van Marken Lichtenbelt WD, Vanhommerig JW, Smulders NM, et al. Cold-activated brown adipose tissue in healthy men. *N Engl J Med*, 2009; 360(15):1500–1508.
6. Xue B, Rim JS, Hogan JC, et al. Genetic variability affects the development of brown adipocytes in white fat but not in interscapular brown fat. *J Lipid Res*, 2007; 48(1):41–51.
7. Rosen ED, MacDougald OA. Adipocyte differentiation from the inside out. *Nat Rev Mol Cell Biol*, 2006 Dec; 7(12):885–896.
8. Spalding KL, Arner E, Westermark PO, et al. Dynamics of fat cell turnover in humans. *Nature*, 2008; 453(7196):783–787.
9. Kienzle E, Zentek J, Meyer H. Body composition of puppies and young dogs. *J Nutr*, 1998; 128(12):2680S–2683S.
10. Alexander LG, Salt C, Thomas G, Butterwick R. Effects of neutering on food intake, body weight and body composition in growing female kittens. *Br J Nutr*, 2011; 106:S19–S23.
11. Kilborn SH, Trudel G, Uhthoff H. Review of growth plate closure compared with age at sexual maturity and lifespan in laboratory animals. *Contemp Top Lab Anim Sci*, 2002 September; 41(5):21–26.
12. Attie AD, Scherer PE. Adipocyte metabolism and obesity. *J Lipid Res*, 2009 Apr; 50:S395–S399.
13. Guilherme A, Virbasius JV, Puri V, Czech MP. Adipocyte dysfunctions linking obesity to insulin resistance and type 2 diabetes. *Nat Rev Mol Cell Biol*, 2008 May; 9(5):367–377.
14. Wozniak SE, Gee LL, Wachtel MS, Frezza EE. Adipose tissue: the new endocrine organ? A review article. *Dig Dis Sci*, 2009 Sep; 54(9):1847–1856.
15. Schäffler A, Schölmerich J, Buechler C. The role of "adipotropins" and the clinical importance of a potential hypothalamic–pituitary–adipose axis. *Nat Clin Pract Endocrinol Metab*, 2006; 2:374–383.
16. Blundell J, de Graaf C, Hulshof T, et al. Appetite control: methodological aspects of the evaluation of foods. *Obes Rev*, 2010 Mar; 11(3): 251–270.
17. Morton GJ, Cummings DE, Baskin DG, et al. Central nervous system control of food intake and body weight. *Nature*, 2006 Sep 21; 443(7109):289–295.
18. D'Alessio DA, Kieffer TJ, Taborsky GJ Jr, Havel PJ. Activation of the parasympathetic nervous system is necessary for normal meal-induced insulin secretion in rhesus macaques. *J Clin Endocrinol Metab*, 2001 Mar; 86(3):1253–1259.
19. Asmar M, Holst JJ. Glucagon-like peptide 1 and glucose-dependent insulinotropic polypeptide: new advances. *Curr Opin Endocrinol Diabetes Obes*, 2010 Feb; 17(1):57–62.
20. Wideman RD, Kieffer TJ. Mining incretin hormone pathways for novel therapies. *Trends Endocrinol Metab*, 2009 Aug; 20(6):280–286.

21. Vahl TP, Drazen DL, Seeley RJ, et al. Meal-anticipatory glucagon-like peptide-1 secretion in rats. *Endocrinology*, 2010 Feb; 151(2):569–575.
22. Turton MD, O'Shea D, Gunn I, et al. A role for glucagon-like peptide-1 in the central regulation of feeding. *Nature*, 1996; 379(6560):69–72.
23. Ahren B, Holst JJ. The cephalic insulin response to meal ingestion in humans is dependent on both cholinergic and noncholinergic mechanisms and is important for postprandial glycemia. *Diabetes*, 2001 May; 50(5):1030–1038.
24. Farilla L, Bulotta A, Hirshberg B, et al. Glucagon-like peptide 1 inhibits cell apoptosis and improves glucose responsiveness of freshly isolated human islets. *Endocrinology*, 2003 Dec; 144(12):5149–5158.
25. de Koning EJ, Bonner-Weir S, Rabelink TJ. Preservation of β-cell function by targeting β-cell mass. *Trends Pharmacol Sci*, 2008 Apr; 29(4):218–227.
26. Chandra R, Liddle RA. Cholecystokinin. *Curr Opin Endocrinol Diabetes Obes*, 2007 Feb; 14(1):63–67.
27. Raybould HE. Mechanisms of CCK signaling from gut to brain. *Curr Opin Pharmacol*, 2007 Dec; 7(6): 570–574.
28. Murphy KG, Dhillo WS, Bloom SR. Gut peptides in the regulation of food intake and energy homeostasis. *Endocr Rev*, 2006 Dec; 27(7):719–727.
29. Wynne K, Bloom SR. The role of oxyntomodulin and peptide tyrosine-tyrosine (PYY) in appetite control. *Nat Clin Pract Endocrinol Metab*, 2006; 2(11):612–620.
30. Cohen MA, Ellis SM, Le Roux CW, et al. Oxyntomodulin suppresses appetite and reduces food intake in humans. *J Clin Endocrinol Metab*, 2003 Oct; 88(10):4696–4701.
31. Wynne K, Park AJ, Small CJ, et al. Oxyntomodulin increases energy expenditure in addition to decreasing energy intake in overweight and obese humans: a randomised controlled trial. *Int J Obes (Lond)*, 2006 Dec; 30(12):1729–1736.
32. Holst JJ, Wewer Albrechtsen NJ, Nordskov Gabe MB, Rosenkilde MM. Oxyntomodulin: Actions and role in diabetes. *Peptides*, 2018; 100:48–53.
33. Pocai A. Action and therapeutic potential of oxyntomodulin. *Mol Metab*, 2014 June; 3(3):241–251.
34. Batterham RL, Cowley MA, Small CJ, et al. Gut hormone PYY(3-36) physiologically inhibits food intake. *Nature*, 2002 Aug 8; 418(6898):650–654.
35. Zwirska-Korczala K, Konturek SJ, Sodowski M, et al. Basal and postprandial plasma levels of PYY, ghrelin, cholecystokinin, gastrin and insulin in women with moderate and morbid obesity and metabolic syndrome. *J Physiol Pharmacol*, 2007; 58(Suppl 1):13–35.
36. Batterham RL, Cohen MA, Ellis SM, et al. Inhibition of food intake in obese subjects by peptide YY3–36. *N Engl J Med*, 2003 Sep 4; 349(10):941–948.
37. Teff KL, Grudziak J, Townsend RR, et al. Endocrine and metabolic effects of consuming fructose-and glucose-sweetened beverages with meals in obese men and women: influence of insulin resistance on plasma triglyceride responses. *J Clin Endocrinol Metab*, 2009 May; 94(5):1562–1569.
38. Elmquist JK, Coppari R, Balthasar N, et al. Identifying hypothalamic pathways controlling food intake, body weight, and glucose homeostasis. *J Comp Neurol*, 2005 Dec 5; 493(1):63–71.
39. Müller TD, Nogueiras R, Andermann ML, et al. Ghrelin. *Mol Metab*, 2015 Jun; 4(6):437–460.
40. Shintani M, Ogawa Y, Ebihara K, et al. Ghrelin, an endogenous growth hormone secretagogue, is a novel orexigenic peptide that antagonizes leptin action through the activation of hypothalamic neuropeptide Y/Y1 receptor pathway. *Diabetes*, 2001 Feb; 50(2):227–232.
41. Erdmann J, Tahbaz R, Lippl F, et al. Plasma ghrelin levels during exercise – effects of intensity and duration. *Regul Pept*, 2007 Oct 4; 143(1–3):127–135.
42. Erdmann J, Töpsch R, Lippl F, et al. Postprandial response of plasma ghrelin levels to various test meals in relation to food intake, plasma insulin, and glucose. *J Clin Endocrinol Metab*, 2004 Jun; 89(6):3048–3054.

43. English PJ, Ghatei MA, Malik IA, et al. Food fails to suppress ghrelin levels in obese humans. *J Clin Endocrinol Metab*, 2002 Jun; 87(6):2984.

44. Purnell JQ, Cummings D, Weigle DS. Changes in 24-h area-under-the-curve ghrelin values following diet-induced weight loss are associated with loss of fat-free mass, but not with changes in fat mass, insulin levels or insulin sensitivity. *Int J Obes (Lond)*, 2007 Feb; 31(2):385–389.

45. Leidy HJ, Gardner JK, Frye BR, et al. Circulating ghrelin is sensitive to changes in body weight during a diet and exercise program in normal-weight young women. *J Clin Endocrinol Metab*, 2004 Jun; 89(6):2659–2664.

46. Daousi C, Wilding JP, Aditya S, et al. Effects of peripheral administration of synthetic human glucose-dependent insulinotropic peptide (GIP) on energy expenditure and subjective appetite sensations in healthy normal weight subjects and obese patients with type 2 diabetes. *Clin Endocrinol (Oxf)*, 2009 Aug; 71(2):195–201.

47. Brunson BL, Zhong Q, Clarke KJ, et al. Serum concentrations of adiponectin and characterization of adiponectin protein complexes in dogs. *Am J Vet Res*, 2007; 68(1):57–62.

48. Zini E, Linscheid P, Franchini M, et al. Partial sequencing and expression of genes involved in glucose metabolism in adipose tissues and skeletal muscle of healthy cats. *Vet J*, 2009; 180(1):66–70.

49. Bergman RN, Kim SP, Catalano KJ, et al. Why visceral fat is bad: mechanisms of the metabolic syndrome. *Obesity (Silver Spring)*, 2006; 14(Suppl 1):16S–19S.

50. Shoelson SE, Lee J, Goldfine AB. Inflammation and insulin resistance *J Clin Invest*, 2006 Jul 3; 116(7):1793–1801.

51. Havel PJ. Update on adipocyte hormones: regulation of energy balance and carbohydrate/lipid metabolism. *Diabetes*, 2004 Feb; 53(Suppl 1):S143–S151.

52. Kubota N, Yano W, Kubota T, et al. Adiponectin stimulates AMP-activated protein kinase in the hypothalamus and increases food intake. *Cell Metab*, 2007 Jul; 6(1):55–68.

53. Park HJ, Lee SE, Oh JH, et al. Leptin, adiponectin and serotonin levels in lean and obese dogs. *BMC Vet Res*, 2014; 10:113.

54. Mazaki-Tovi M, Abood SK, Segev G, Schenck PA. Alterations in adipokines in feline hepatic lipidosis. *J Vet Intern Med*, 2013 Mar–Apr; 27(2):242–249.

55. Bjornvad CR, Rand JS, Tan HY, et al. Obesity and sex influence insulin resistance and total and multimer adiponectin levels in adult neutered domestic shorthair client-owned cats. *Domest Anim Endocrinol*, 2014 Apr; 47:55–64.

56. Ishioka K, Omachi A, Sasaki N, et al. Feline adiponectin: molecular structures and plasma concentrations in obese cats. *J Vet Med Sci*, 2009 Feb; 71(2):189–194.

57. Lee B, Shao J. Adiponectin and energy homeostasis. *Rev Endocr Metab Disord*, 2014 Jun; 15(2):149–156.

58. Ishioka K, Omachi A, Sagawa M, et al. Canine adiponectin: cDNA structure, mRNA expression adipose tissues and reduced plasma levels in obesity. *Res Vet Sci*, 2006; 80(2):127–132.

59. Neschen S, Morino K, Rossbacher JC, et al. Fish oil regulates adiponectin secretion by a peroxisome proliferator-activated receptor-gamma-dependent mechanism in mice. *Diabetes*, 2006; 55(4):924–928.

60. Rossi AS, Lombardo YB, Lacorte JM, et al. Dietary fish oil positively regulates plasma leptin and adiponectin levels in sucrose-fed, insulin-resistant rats. *Am J Physiol Regul Integr Comp Physiol*, 2005; 289(2):486–494.

61. Ishioka K, Soliman MM, Sagawa M, et al. Experimental and clinical studies on plasma leptin in obese dogs. *J Vet Med Sci*, 2002; 64(4):349–353.

62. Backus RC, Havel PJ, Gingerich RL, Rogers QR. Relationship between serum leptin immunoreactivity and body fat mass as estimated by use of a novel gas-phase Fourier transform infrared spectroscopy deuterium dilution method in cats. *Am J Vet Res*, 2000; 61(7):796–801.

63. Appleton DJ, Rand JS, Sunvold GD. Plasma leptin concentrations in cats: reference range, effect of weight gain and relationship with adiposity as measured by dual energy X-ray absorptiometry. *J Feline Med Surg*, 2000; 2(4):191–199.

64. Martin LJ, Siliart B, Dumon H, et al. Leptin, body fat content and energy expenditure in intact and gonadectomized adult cats: a preliminary study. *J Anim Physiol Anim Nutr*, 2001; 85(7–8):195–199.

65. Park HK, Ahima RS. Physiology of leptin: energy homeostasis, neuroendocrine function and metabolism. *Metabolism*, 2015 Jan; 64(1):24–34.

66. Ishioka K, Hosoya K, Kitagawa H, et al. Plasma leptin concentration in dogs: effects of body condition score, age, gender, and breeds. *Res Vet Sci*, 2007; 82(1):11–15.

67. Martin LJ, Siliart B, Dumon HJ, Nguyen P. Spontaneous hormonal variations in male cats following gonadectomy. *J Feline Med Surg*, 2006; 8(5):309–314.

68. Belsito KR, Vester BM, Keel T, et al. Impact of ovariohysterectomy and food intake on body composition, physical activity, and adipose gene expression in cats. *J Anim Sci*, 2009; 87(2):594–602.

69. Friedman JM. The alphabet of weight control. *Nature*, 1997 Jan 9; 385(6612):119–120.

70. Ahima RS, Flier JS. Leptin. *Annu Rev Physiol*, 2000; 62:413–37.

71. Nishii N, Nodake H, Takasu M, et al. Postprandial changes in leptin concentration of cerebrospinal fluid in dogs during development of obesity. *Am J Vet Res*, 2006; 67(12):2006–2011.

72. Chen K, Li F, Li J, et al. Induction of leptin resistance through direct interaction of C-reactive protein with leptin. *Nat Med*, 2006 Apr; 12(4):425–432.

73. Seeley RJ, York DA. Fuel sensing and the central nervous system (CNS): implications for the regulation of energy balance and the treatment for obesity. *Obes Rev*, 2005 Aug; 6(3):259–265.

74. Woods SC. Signals that influence food intake and body weight. *Physiol Behav*, 2005 Dec 15; 86(5):709–716.

75. Seeley RJ, Drazen DL, Clegg DJ. The critical role of the melanocortin system in the control of energy balance. *Annu Rev Nutr*, 2004; 24:133–149.

76. Cone RD. Anatomy and regulation of the central melanocortin system. *Nat Neurosci*, 2005 May; 8(5):571–578.

77. Lee YS, Challis BG, Thompson DA, et al. A POMC variant implicates β-melanocyte-stimulating hormone in the control of human energy balance. *Cell Metab*, 2006 Feb; 3(2):135–140.

78. Cowley MA, Smart JL, Rubinstein M, et al. Leptin activates anorexigenic POMC neurons through a neural network in the arcuate nucleus. *Nature*, 2001 May 24; 411(6836):480–184.

79. Bates SH, Myers MG Jr. The role of leptin receptor signaling in feeding and neuroendocrine function. *Trends Endocrinol Metab*, 2003 Dec; 14(10):447–452.

80. Luquet S, Perez FA, Hnasko TS, Palmiter RD. NPY/AgRP neurons are essential for feeding in adult mice but can be ablated in neonates. *Science*, 2005 Oct 28; 310(5748):683–685.

81. Bellinger LL, Bernardis LL. The dorsomedial hypothalamic nucleus and its role in ingestive behavior and body weight regulation: lessons learned from lesioning studies. *Physiol Behav*, 2002 Jul; 76(3):431–442.

82. Chou TC, Scammell TE, Gooley JJ, et al. Critical role of dorsomedial hypothalamic nucleus in a wide range of behavioral circadian rhythms. *J Neurosci*, 2003 Nov 19; 23(33):10691–10702.

83. Gooley JJ, Schomer A, Saper CB. The dorsomedial hypothalamic nucleus is critical for the expression of food-entrainable circadian rhythms. *Nat Neurosci*, 2006 Mar; 9(3):398–407.

84. Guan JL, Uehara K, Lu S, et al. Reciprocal synaptic relationships between orexin- and melanin-concentrating hormone-containing neurons in the rat lateral hypothalamus: a novel circuit implicated in feeding regulation. *Int J Obes Relat Metab Disord*, 2002 Dec; 26(12):1523–1532.

85. Sahu A. Interactions of neuropeptide Y, hypocretin-I (orexin A) and melanin-concentrating hormone on feeding in rats. *Brain Res*, 2002 Jul 19; 944(1–2):232–238.
86. Kennedy AR, Todd JF, Stanley SA, et al. Melanin-concentrating hormone (MCH) suppresses thyroid stimulating hormone (TSH) release, in vivo and in vitro, via the hypothalamus and the pituitary. *Endocrinology*, 2001 Jul; 142(7):3265–3268.
87. Willie JT, Chemelli RM, Sinton CM, Yanagisawa M. To eat or to sleep? Orexin in the regulation of feeding and wakefulness. *Annu Rev Neurosci*, 2001; 24:429–458.
88. Wise RA. Dopamine, learning and motivation. *Nat Rev Neurosci*, 2004 Jun; 5(6):483–494.
89. Volkow ND, Wise RA. How can drug addiction help us understand obesity? *Nat Neurosci*, 2005 May; 8(5):555–560.
90. Small DM, Jones-Gotman M, Dagher A. Feeding-induced dopamine release in dorsal striatum correlates with meal pleasantness ratings in healthy human volunteers. *Neuroimage*, 2003 Aug; 19(4):1709–1715.
91. Hanley NR, Van de Kar LD. Serotonin and the neuroendocrine regulation of the hypothalamic–pituitary–adrenal axis in health and disease. *Vitam Horm*, 2003; 66:189–255.
92. Stunes AK, Reseland JE, Hauso O, et al. Adipocytes express a functional system for serotonin synthesis, reuptake and receptor activation. *Diabetes Obes Metab*, 2011; 13(6):551–558.
93. Aronne LJ, Thornton-Jones ZD. New targets for obesity pharmacotherapy. *Clin Pharmacol Ther*, 2007; 81(5):748–752.
94. Hill JO, Wyatt HR, Reed GW, Peters JC. Obesity and the environment: where do we go from here? *Science*, 2003 Feb 7; 299(5608):853–855.
95. Elices-Minguez R. Food "extra". In: *Practical atlas of nutrition and feeding in cats and dogs* Volume I. Zaragoza, Spain: Editorial Servet, 2017; pp. 76–77.
96. Karpe F, Fielding BA, Ilic V, et al. Monitoring adipose tissue blood flow in man: a comparison between the (133)xenon washout method and microdialysis. *Int J Obes Relat Metab Disord*, 2002 Jan; 26(1):1–5.
97. Trayhurn P, Wang B, Wood IS. Hypoxia and the endocrine and signalling role of white adipose tissue. *Arch Physiol Biochem*, 2008 Oct; 114(4):267–276.
98. Trayhurn P, Wang B, Wood IS. Hypoxia in adipose tissue: a basis for the dysregulation of tissue function in obesity? *Br J Nutr*, 2008 Aug; 100(2):227–235.
99. Di Girolamo M, Skinner NS Jr, Hanley HG, Sachs RG. Relationship of adipose tissue blood flow to fat cell size and number. *Am J Physiol*, 1971 Apr; 220(4):932–937.
100. Maury E, Brichard SM. Adipokine dysregulation, adipose tissue inflammation and metabolic syndrome. *Mol Cell Endocrinol*, 2010; 314(1):1–16.
101. Jordan ET, Kley S, Le NA, et al. Dyslipidemia in obese cats. *Domest Anim Endocrinol*, 2008; 35(3):290–299.
102. Gayet C, Bailhache E, Dumon H, et al. Insulin resistance and changes in plasma concentrations of TNFα, IGF1, and NEFA in dogs during weight gain and obesity. *J Anim Physiol Anim Nutr*, 2004; 88(3–4):157–165.
103. Boden G. Obesity and Free Fatty Acids (FFA). *Endocrinol Metab Clin North Am*, 2008 Sep; 37(3):635–646.
104. Boden G. Free fatty acids-the link between obesity and insulin resistance. *Endocr Pract*, 2001 Jan–Feb; 7(1):44–51.
105. Schönfeld P, Wojtczak L. Fatty acids as modulators of the cellular production of reactive oxygen species. *Free Radic Biol Med*, 2008 Aug 1; 45(3):231–241.
106. Jerico M, Leonardi A, Pereira V, et al. Clinical evaluation of obese dogs. *31st World Small Animal Veterinary Association World Congress Proceedings*. Czech. Republic, Oct. 11–14, 2006.
107. Clark MH, Larsen R, Lu W, Hoenig M. Investigation of 1H MRS for quantification of hepatic triglyceride in lean and obese cats. *Res Vet Sci*, 2013, 95(2):678–680.
108. Appleton DJ, Rand JS, Sunvold GD. Plasma leptin concentrations are independently associated with insulin sensitivity in lean and overweight cats. *J Feline Med Surg*, 2002; 4(2):83–93.

109. Hoenig M, Thomaseth K, Waldron M, Ferguson DC. Insulin sensitivity, fat distribution and adipocytokine response to different diets in lean and obese cats before and after weight loss. *Am J Physiol*, 2007; 292(1):R227–R234.

110. Chastain CB, Panciera D. Insulin sensitivity decreases with obesity, and lean cats with low insulin sensitivity are at greatest risk of glucose intolerance with weight gain. *Small Anim Clin Endocrinol*, 2002; 12(2):9–10.

111. Haring T, Haase B, Zini E, et al. Overweight and impaired insulin sensitivity present in growing cats. *J Anim Physiol Anim Nutr (Berl)*, 2013; 97(5):813–819.

112. Bailhache E, Nguyen P, Krempf M, et al. Lipoproteins abnormalities in obese insulin-resistant dogs. *Metabolism*, 2003 May; 52(5):559–564.

113. Mattheuws D, Rottiers R, Baeyens D, Vermeulen A. Glucose tolerance and insulin response in obese dogs. *J Am Anim Hosp Assoc*, 1984; 20:287–293.

114. Ferguson DC, Caffall Z, Hoenig M. Obesity increases free thyroxine proportionally to nonesterified fatty acid concentrations in adult neutered female cats. *J Endocrinol*, 2007; 194(2):267–273.

115. Daminet S, Jeusette I, Duchateau L, et al. Evaluation of thyroid function in obese dogs and in dogs undergoing a weight loss protocol. *J Vet Med A Physiol Pathol Clin Med*, 2003; 50(4):213–218.

116. Martin LJ, Siliart B, Dumon HJ, Nguyen PG. Hormonal disturbances associated with obesity in dogs. *J Anim Physiol Anim Nutr (Berl)*, 2006 Oct; 90(9–10):355–360.

117. Yin X, Lanza IR, Swain JM, et al. Adipocyte mitochondrial function is reduced in human obesity independent of fat cell size. *J Clin Endocrinol Metab*, 2014 Feb; 99(2):E209–E216.

118. Karpe F, Dickmann JR, Frayn KN. Fatty acids, obesity, and insulin resistance: time for a reevaluation. *Diabetes*, 2011 Oct; 60(10):2441–2449.

119. Jeusette IC, Lhoest ET, Istasse LP, et al. Influence of obesity on plasma lipid and lipoprotein concentrations in dogs. *Am J Vet Res*, 2005; 66(1):81–86.

120. Tvarijonaviciute A, Ceron JJ, de Torre C, et al. Obese dogs with and without obesity-related metabolic dysfunction – a proteomic approach. *BMC Vet Res*, 2016 Sep 20; 12:211.

121. Tvarijonaviciute A, Ceron JJ, Holden SL, et al. Obesity-related metabolic dysfunction in dogs: a comparison with human metabolic syndrome. *BMC Vet Res*, 2012; 8:147.

122. Després JP, Lemieux I. Abdominal obesity and metabolic syndrome. *Nature*, 2006 December 14; 444(7121):881–887.

123. Even SE, Rios FJ, Dinh Cat AN, et al. Adipocyte-derived aldosterone and cortisol are Nox1/4 dependent: implications in obesity-associated vascular dysfunction. *Hypertension*. 2014; 64:A010.

124. Spencer SJ. Early life programming of obesity: the impact of the perinatal environment on the development of obesity and metabolic dysfunction in the offspring. *Curr Diabetes Rev*, 2012 Jan; 8(1):55–68.

125. Sun X, Morris KL, Zemel MB. Role of calcitriol and cortisol on human adipocyte proliferation and oxidative and inflammatory stress: a microarray study. *J Nutrigenet Nutrigenomics*, 2008; 1(1–2):30–48.

126. Wenger RH. Cellular adaptation to hypoxia: O_2-sensing protein hydroxylases, hypoxia-inducible transcription factors, and O_2-regulated gene expression. *FASEB J*, 2002 Aug; 16(10):1151–1162.

127. Sallander M, Eliasson J, Hedhammar A. Prevalence and risk factors for the development of diabetes mellitus in Swedish cats. *Acta Vet Scand*, 2012; 54:61.

128. Prahl A, Guptill L, Glickman NW, et al. Time trends and risk factors for diabetes mellitus in cats presented to veterinary teaching hospitals. *J Feline Med Surg*, 2007; 9(5):351–358.

129. O'Neill DG, Gostelow R, Orme C, et al. Epidemiology of diabetes mellitus among 193,435 cats attending primary-care veterinary practices in England. *J Vet Intern Med*, 2016 Jul; 30(4):964–972.

130. Hoenig M, Pach N, Thomaseth K, et al. Cats differ from other species in their cytokine and antioxidant enzyme response when developing obesity. *Obesity (Silver Spring)*, 2013; 21:E407–E414.

131. Forcada Y, Holder AL, Church DB, Catchpole B. A polymorphism in the melanocortin 4 receptor gene (MC4R:c.92C>T) is associated with diabetes mellitus in overweight domestic shorthaired cats. *J Vet Intern Med*, 2014; 28(2):458–464.

132. Forcada Y, Boursnell M, Catchpole B, Church DB. A genome-wide association study identifies novel candidate genes for the susceptibility to diabetes mellitus in DSH cats [abstract]. *25th ECVIM-CA Congress*, 2015 Sep 10–12; Lisbon, Portugal.

133. Hay DL, Chen S, Lutz TA, et al. Amylin: pharmacology, physiology, and clinical potential. *Pharmacol Rev*, 2015 Jul; 67(3):564–600.

134. Lutz TA. Feline diabetes mellitus: nutritional strategies. In: Pibot P, Biourge V, Elliott D. *Encyclopedia of Feline Clinical Nutrition*. Aimargues, France: Aniwa SAS on behalf of Royal Canin, 2008; pp. 181–222.

135. Rand JS. Pathogenesis of feline diabetes. *Vet Clin North Am Small Anim Pract*, 2013 Mar; 43(2):221–231.

136. Bjornvad CR, Rand JS, Tan HY, et al. Obesity and sex influence insulin resistance and total and multimer adiponectin levels in adult neutered domestic shorthair client-owned cats. *Domest Anim Endocrinol*, 2014 Apr; 47(1):55–64.

137. Lee P, Mori A, Coradini M, et al. Potential predictive biomarkers of obesity in Burmese cats. *Vet J*, 2013; 195(2):221–227.

Chapter 3. Identification and evaluation of obese patients

1. Kealy RD, Lawler DF, Ballam JM, et al. Effects of diet restriction on life span and age-related changes in dogs. *J Am Vet Med Assoc*, 2002 May 1; 220(9):1315–1320.

2. Lawler DF, Evans RH, Larson BT, et al. Influence of lifetime food restriction on causes, time, and predictors of death in dogs. *J Am Vet Med Assoc*, 2005 Jan 15; 226(2):225–231.

3. Speakman JR, Booles D, Butterwick R. Validation of dual energy X-ray absorptiometry (DXA) by comparison with chemical analysis of dogs and cats. *Int J Obes Relat Metab Disord*, 2001; 25:439–447.

4. Jeusette I, Greco D, Aquino F, et al. Effect of breed on body composition and comparison between various methods to estimate body composition in dogs. *Res Vet Sci*, 2010 Apr; 88(2):227–232.

5. Lauten SD, Cox NR, Brawner Jr WR, Baker HJ. Use of dual energy X-ray absorptiometry for noninvasive body composition measurements in clinically normal dogs. *Am J Vet Res*, 2001; 62(8):1295–1301.

6. Speakman JR, van Acker A, Harper EJ. Age-related changes in the metabolism and body composition of three dog breeds and their relationship to life expectancy. *Aging Cell*, 2003; 2(5):265–275.

7. Laflamme, D. Development and validation of a body condition score system for dogs. *Canine Pract*, 1997; 22(4):10–15.

8. Laflamme D. Development and validation of a body condition score system for cats: a clinical tool. *Feline Pract*, 1997; 25(5):13–18.

9. Wilkinson MJ, McEwan NA. Use of ultrasound in the measurement of subcutaneous fat and prediction of total body fat in dogs. *J Nutr*, 1991; 121(11 Suppl):S4—S50.

10. Bjornvad CR, Nielsen DH, Armstrong PJ, et al. Evaluation of a nine-point body condition scoring system in physically inactive pet cats. *Am J Vet Res*, 2011 April; 72(4):433–437.

11. Scott KC, Levy JK, Gorman SP, Newell SM. Body condition of feral cats and the effect of neutering. *J Appl Anim Welf Sci*, 2002; 5(3):203–213.

12. Laflamme DP, Kealy RD, Schmidt DA. Estimation of body fat by body condition score. *J Vet Int Med*, 1994; 8:154.

13. Raffan E, Holden SL, Cullingham F, et al. Standardized positioning is essential for precise determination of body composition using dual-energy X-ray absorptiometry in dogs. *J Nutr*, 2006; 136(7):1976S–1978S.

14. Munday HS, Booles D, Anderson P, et al. The repeatability of body condition measurements in dogs and cats using dual energy X-ray absorptiometry. *J. Nutr*, 1994; 124:2619S-2621S.

15. Hendriks WH, Moughan PJ, Tarttelin MF. Body composition of the adult domestic cat (*Felis catus*). *J Anim Physiol Anim Nutr (Berl)*, 1996; 77:16—23.

16. Witzel AL, Kirk CA, Henry GA, et al. Use of a novel morphometric method and body fat index system for estimation of body composition in overweight and obese dogs. *J Am Vet Med Assoc*, 2014; 244(11):1279–1284.
17. Meyer H, Drochner W, Weidenhaupt C. Ein beitrag zum vorkommen und der behandluny der adipositas des hundes. [A contribution to the occurrence and treatment of obesity in dogs]. *Dtsch Tierarztl Wochenschr*, 1978; 85(4):133–136.
18. Krook L, Larsson S, Rooney JR. The interrelationship of diabetes mellitus, obesity, and pyometra in the dog. *Am J Vet Res*, 1960; 21:120–127.
19. Drost WT, Couto CG, Fischetti AJ, et al. Comparison of glomerular filtration rate between greyhounds and non-Greyhound dogs. *J Vet Intern Med*, 2006; 20(3):544–546.
20. Jackson AS, Stanforth PR, Gagnon J, et al. The effect of sex, age and race on estimating percentage body fat from body mass index: The Heritage Family Study. *Int J Obes Relat Metab Disord*, 2002; 26(6):789–796.
21. Kienzle E, Stratmann B, Meyer H. Body composition of cats as a basis for factorial calculation of energy and nutrient requirements for growth. *J Nutr*, 1991; 121(11 Suppl):S122 S123.
22. Kienzle E, Zentek J, Meyer H. Body composition of puppies and young dogs. *J Nutr*, 1998 Dec; 128(12 Suppl):2680S–2683S.
23. Burkholder WJ, Thatcher CD. Validation of predictive equations for use of deuterium oxide dilution to determine body composition of dogs. *Am J Vet Res*, 1998; 59(8):927–937.
24. Son HR, d'Avignon DA, Laflamme DP. Comparison of dual-energy X-ray absorptiometry and measurement of total body water content by deuterium oxide dilution for estimating body composition in dogs. *Am J Vet Res*, 1998 May; 59(5):529–532.
25. Sagawa M, Yoneda S, Nakadomo F. Kinetics of deuterium in dogs following intravenous administration of deuterium oxide. The primary study for measurement of canine body fat mass by deuterium oxide dilution method. *J Pet Anim Nutr*, 2000; 3(2):67–71.
26. Ferrier L, Robert P, Dumon H, et al. Evaluation of body composition in dogs by isotopic dilution using a low-cost technique, Fourier-transform infrared spectroscopy. *J Nutr*, 2002 June 1; 132(6 Suppl 2):1725S–1727S.
27. Madsen OR, Jensen JEB, Sorensen OH. Validation of a dual energy X-ray absorptiometer: measurement of bone mass and soft tissue composition. *Eur J Appl Physiol Occup Physiol*, 1997; 75(6):554–558.
28. Mawby DI, Bartges JW, d'Avignon A, et al. Comparison of various methods for estimating body fat in dogs. *J Am Anim Hosp Assoc*, 2004; 40(2):109–114.
29. Borges NC, Vasconcellos RS, Carciofi AC, et al. DXA, bioelectrical impedance, ultrasonography and biometry for the estimation of fat and lean mass in cats during weight loss. *BMC Vet Res*, 2012; 8(1):111.
30. Jebb SA, Goldberg G, Jennings G, Elia M. Dual-energy X-ray absorptiometry measurements of body composition: effects of depth and tissue thickness, including comparisons with direct analysis. *Clin Sci (Lond)*, 1995; 88(3):319–324.
31. Ishioka K, Okumura M, Sagawa M, et al. Computed tomographic assessment of body fat in beagles. *Vet Radiol Ultrasound*, 2005; 46(1):49–53.
32. Purushothaman D, Vanselow BA, Wu SB, et al. Whole body computed tomography with advanced imaging techniques: a research tool for measuring body composition in dogs. *J Vet Med*, 2013; 2013:610654.
33. Stone R, Berghoff N, Steiner JM, Zoran D. Use of a bioelectric impedance device in obese and lean healthy dogs to estimate body fat percentage. *Vet Ther*, 2009; 10(1–2):59–70.
34. Thomas BJ, Ward LC, Cornish BH. Bioimpedance spectrometry in the determination of body water compartments: Accuracy and clinical significance. *Appl Radiat Isot*, 1998; 49:447–455.
35. Stanton CA, Hamar DW, Johnson DE, Fettman MJ. Bioelectrical impedance and zoometry for body composition analysis in domestic cats. *Am J Vet Res*, 1992; 53(2):251–257.

36. Rae LS, Vankan DM, Rand JS, et al. Measuring body composition in dogs using multifrequency bioelectrical impedance analysis and dual energy X-ray absorptiometry. *Vet J*, 2016; 212:65–70.

37. Yaguiyan-Colliard L, Daumas C, Bousbiat S, et al. Indirect assessment of total body water in adult beagle dogs by single-frequency bioelectrical impedance analysis (SF-BIA). *Am J Vet Res*, 2015; 76(6):547–553.

38. Yaguiyan-Colliard L, Daumas C, Nguyen P, et al. Evaluation of total body water in canine breeds by single-frequency bioelectrical impedance analysis method: specific equations are needed for accuracy. *BMC Res Notes*, 2015 8:336.

39. Elliott DA, Backus RC, Van Loan MD, Rogers QR. Extracellular water and total body water estimated by multifrequency bioelectrical impedance analysis in healthy cats: a cross-validation study. *J. Nutr*, 2002; 132(6 Suppl 2):1760S–1762S.

40. Morooka T, Niiyama M, Uchida E, et al. Measurement of the back fat layer in beagles for estimation of obesity using two-dimensional ultrasonography. *J Small Anim Pract*, 2001; 42(2):56–59.

41. Yamka RM, Friesen KG, Stiers CA, et al. Using ultrasound as an alternative method for determining body fat in beagles. *J Anim Sci*, 2007; 85(Suppl 1):266.

42. Payan-Carreira R, Martins L, Miranda S, et al. In vivo assessment of subcutaneous fat in dogs by real-time ultrasonography and image analysis. *Acta Vet Scand*, 2016; 58(Suppl 1):58.

43. Hawthorne AJ, Butterwick RF. The feline body mass index – a simple measure of body fat content in cats. *WALTHAM Focus*, 2000; 10(1):32–33.

44. Laflamme DP, Hume E, Harrison J. Evaluation of zoometric measures as an assessment of body composition of dogs and cats. *Compend Contin Educ Pract Vet*, 2001; 23(Suppl 9A):88.

45. Burkholder WJ. *Body composition of dogs determined by carcass composition analysis, deuterium oxide dilution, subjective and objective morphometry, and bioelectrical impedance* (PhD Dissertation). Blacksburg, VA: Virginia Polytechnic Institute and State University, 1994.

46. Witzel AL, Kirk CA, Henry GA, et al. Use of a morphometric method and body fat index system for estimation of body composition in overweight and obese cats. *J Am Vet Med Assoc*, 2014; 244(11):1285–1290.

47. Elices-Minguez R. Body score system; Morphometric measurements. In: *Practical atlas of nutrition and feeding in cats and dogs* Volume I. Zaragoza, Spain: Servet Editorial, 2017; pp. 10–13.

48. Committee on Dog and Cat Nutrition, National Research Council. *Nutrient requirements of dogs and cats*. Washington, DC: National Academies Press. 2006.

49. Edney AT, Smith PM. Study of obesity in dogs visiting veterinary practices in the United Kingdom. *Vet Rec*, 1986; 118(14):391–396.

50. Bjornvad CR, Nielsen DH, Armstrong PJ, et al. Evaluation of a nine-point body condition scoring system in physically inactive pet cats. *Am J Vet Res*, 2011; 72(4):433–437.

51. Burkholder WJ. Use of body condition scores in clinical assessment of the provision of optimal nutrition. *J Am Vet Med Assoc*, 2000; 217(5):650–654.

52. Yamka RM, Friesen KG, Frantz NZ. Identification of canine markers related to obesity and the effects of weight loss on the markers of interest. *Intern J Appl Res Vet Med*, 2006; 4(4):282–292.

53. Yamka RM, Friesen KG. Identification of markers related to feline obesity. *J Anim Sci*, 2006; 84(Suppl 1):171–172.

54. AOAC. *Official Methods of Analysis of AOAC International*, 20th Edition. 2016. www.aoac.org.

Chapter 4. Communication with owners

1. American Animal Hospital Association. *The path to high-quality care. Practical tips for improving compliance.* Denver (CO): American Animal Hospital Association; 2003.
2. *Ley 4/2016, de 22 de julio, de Protección de los Animales de Compañía de la Comunidad de Madrid.* BOCM 10 de agosto de 2016. BOE 25 de noviembre de 2016.
3. Kealy RD, Lawler DF, Ballam JM, et al. 2002. Effects of diet restriction on life span and age-related changes in dogs. *J Am Vet Med Assoc*, 2002; May 1; 220(9):1315–1320.
4. World Health Organization. *Adherence to long-term therapies: evidence for action.* Geneva (Switzerland): WHO Library Cataloguing, 2003.
5. Prochaska, JO, DiClemente, CC. Transtheoretical therapy: toward a more integrative model of change. *Psychother Theory Res Pract*, 1982; 19:276–288.
6. Keller VF, Carroll JG. A new model for physician-patient communication. *Patient Educ Couns*, 1994; 23(2):131–140.
7. Frankel RM, Stein TS. *The four habits of highly effective clinicians: a practical guide.* Kaiser Permanente Northern California Region, Oakland (CA): Physician Education and Development, 1996.
8. Carroll, JG, Goldstein, MG. Difficult patients or relationships. *AAOS Bulletin*, 2003 Oct. http://www2.aaos.org/bulletin/oct03/comm.htm.
9. Pichert JW, Miller CS, Hollo AH, et al. What health professionals can do to identify and resolve patient dissatisfaction. *Jt Comm J Qual Improv*, 1998; 24(6):303–312.
10. Pease A, Pease B. *The definitive book of body language.* New York City: Bantam Books, 2006.
11. Carson C. Nonverbal communication. In: Cole S, Bird J (eds.). *The medical interview: the three-function approach.* Philadelphia: Mosby; 2000. pp. 225–238.
12. Shaw J, Adams CL, Bonnett BN, et al. Use of the roter interaction analysis system to analyze veterinary-client-patient communication in companion animal practice. *J Am Vet Med Assoc*, 2004; 225(2):222–229.
13. Wayner CJ, Heinke ML. Compliance: crafting quality care. *Vet Clin North Am Small Anim Pract*, 2006; 36(2):419–436.
14. White, GA, Hobson-West P, Cobb K, et al. Canine obesity: is there a difference between veterinarian and owner perception? *J Small Anim Pract*, 2011 Dec; 52(12):622–626.
15. Colliard L, Ancel J, Benet JJ, et al. Risk factors for obesity in dogs in France. *J Nutr*, 2006 Jul; 136(7 Suppl):1951S–1954S.
16. Kienzle E, Bergler R, Mandernach A. A comparison of the feeding behavior and the human-animal relationship in owners of normal and obese dogs. *J Nutr*, 1998 Dec; 128(12 Suppl):2779S–2782S.
17. Singh R, Laflamme P, Sidebottom-Nielsen M. Owner perceptions of canine body condition score. *J Vet Intern Med*, 2002; 16:362.
18. Colliard L, Paragon BM, Lemuet B, et al. Prevalence and risk factors of obesity in an urban population of healthy cats. *J Feline Med Surg*, 2009 Feb; 11(2):135–140.
19. Kienzle E, Bergler R. Human-animal relationship of owners of normal and overweight cats. *J Nutr*, 2006 Jul; 136(7 Suppl):1947S–1950S.
20. Parry LL, Netuveli G, Parry J, Saxena S. A systematic review of parental perception of overweight status in children. *J Ambul Care Manage*, 2008 Jul-Sep; 31(3):253–268.
21. He M, Evans A. Are parents aware that their children are overweight or obese? Do they care? *Can Fam Physician*, 2007 Sep, 53(9):1493–1499.
22. Baker DW, Gazmararian JA, Sudano J, Patterson M. The association between age and health literacy among elderly persons. *J Gerontol B Psychol Sci Soc Sci*, 2000; 55(6):S368–S374.

Chapter 5. Nutrients in weight-loss programmes

1. Evans H, de Lahunta A. *Miller's Anatomy of the dog*. 4th edition. Philadelphia: Saunders, 2013.
2. Grandage J. Functional anatomy of the digestive system. Section 5, Chapter 35:499. In: Slatter, D. (ed.), *Textbook of small animal surgery*. 3rd edition. Philadelphia: Saunders, 2003.
3. *Regulation (EC) No 767/2009 of the European Parliament and of the Council of 13 July 2009 on the placing on the market and use of feed.*
4. *Commission Directive 2008/38/EC of 5 March 2008 establishing a list of intended uses of animal feedingstuffs for particular nutritional purposes.*
5. FEDIAF (Fédération Européenne de l'Industrie des Aliments pour Animaux Familiers). *Nutritional guidelines for complete and complementary pet food for cats and dogs*. Official Publication, July 2016. http://www.fediaf.org/
6. AAFCO (Association of American Feed Control Officials). *Official Publication*, 2014. http://www.aafco.org/
7. Borne AT, Wolfsheimer KJ, Truett AA, et al. Differential metabolic effects of energy restriction in dogs using diets varying in fat and fiber content. *Obes Res*, 1996; 4(4):337–345.
8. Sacks FM, Bray GA, Carey VJ, et al. Comparison of weight-loss diets with different compositions of fat, protein, and carbohydrates. *N Engl J Med*, 2009, Feb 26; 360(9):859–873.
9. Turner-McGrievy GM, Barnard ND, Scialli AR. A two-year randomized weight loss trial comparing a vegan diet to a more moderate low-fat diet. *Obesity (Silver Spring)*, 2007; 15(9):2276–2281.
10. Toll PW, Yamka RM, Schoenherr WD, Hand MS. Chapter 27, Obesity. In: Hand, et al. (eds.), *Small Animal Clinical Nutrition*. 5th edition. Topeka (KS): Mark Morris Institute, 2010.
11. NRC (National Research Council). Subcommittee on Dog and Cat Nutrition, Committee on Animal Nutrition. *Nutrient Requirements of Dogs and Cats*. Washington, DC: The National Academies Press, 2006.
12. Serhan CH. Novel chemical mediators in the resolution of inflammation: resolvins and protectins. *Anesthesiol Clin*, 2006; 24(2):341–364.
13. Chung MY, Yeung SF, Park HJ, et al. Dietary α- and γ-tocopherol supplementation attenuates lipopolysaccharide-induced oxidative stress and inflammatory-related responses in an obese mouse model of nonalcoholic steatohepatitis. *J Nutr Biochem*, 2010; 21(12):1200–1206.
14. Tanner AE, Martin J, Thatcher CD, et al. Nutritional amelioration of oxidative stress induced by obesity and acute weight loss. *Comp Cont Ed Pract Vet*, 2006; 28(Suppl. 4):72.
15. Vajro P, Mandato C, Franzese A, et al. Vitamin E treatment in pediatric obesity-related liver disease: a randomized study. *J Pediatr Gastroenterol Nutr*, 2004; 38(1):48–55.
16. Liu Q, Bengmark S, Qu S. The role of hepatic fat accumulation in pathogenesis of non-alcoholic fatty liver disese (NAFLD). *Lipids Health Dis*, 2010; 9(1):42.
17. Jericó M, Leonardi A, Pereira V, et al. Clinical evaluation of obese dogs. 3*1st World Small Animal Veterinary Association World Congress Proceedings*. Czech. Republic, Oct. 11–14, 2006.
18. Hendriks WH, Wu YB, Shields RG, et al. Vitamin E requirement of adult cats increases slightly with high dietary intake of polyunsaturated fatty acids. *J Nutr*, 2002; 132:1613S–1615S.
19. Hall JA. Potential adverse effects of long-term consumption of (n-3) fatty acids. *Comp Cont Ed Pract Vet*, 1996; 18(8):879–895.
20. Fekete S, Hullar I, Andrasofszky E, et al. Reduction of the energy density of cat foods by increasing their fibre content with a view to nutrients' digestibility. *J Anim Physiol Anim Nutr (Berl)*, 2001; 85(7-8):200–204.
21. Kritchevsky D. Dietary fiber in health and disease. In: *Advanced dietary fibre technology*. Oxford, UK: Blackwell Science, 2001; p. 151.

22. Fahey GC Jr, Merchen NR, Corbin JE, et al. Dietary fiber for dogs: II. Iso-total dietary fiber (TDF) additions of divergent fiber sources to dog diets and their effects on nutrient intake, digestibility, metabolizable energy and digesta mean retention time. *J Anim Sci*, 1990; 68(12):4229–4235.
23. Fahey GC Jr, Merchen NR, Corbin JE, et al. Dietary fiber for dogs: I. Effects of graded levels of dietary beet pulp on nutrient intake, digestibility, metabolizable energy and digesta mean retention time. *J Anim Sci*, 1990; 68(12):4221–4228.
24. Jewell DE, Toll PW, Novotny BJ. Satiety reduces adiposity in dogs. *Vet Ther*, 2000; 1(1):17–23.
25. Bosch G, Verbrugghe A, Hesta M, et al. The effects of dietary fibre type on satiety-related hormones and voluntary food intake in dogs. *Br J Nutr*, 2009; 102(2):318–325.
26. Butterwick RF, Markwell PJ, Thorne CJ. Effect of level and source of dietary fiber on food intake in the dog. *J Nutr*, 1994; 124(12):2695S–2700S.
27. Jewell DE, Toll PW. Effects of fiber on food intake in dogs. *Vet Clin Nutr*, 1996; 3:115–118.
28. Jackson JR, Laflamme DP, Owens SF. Effects of dietary fiber content on satiety in dogs. *Vet Clin Nutr*, 1997; 4:130–134.
29. Butterwick RF, Markwell PJ. Effect of amount and type of dietary fiber on food intake in energy-restricted dogs. *Am J Vet Res*, 1997; 58(3):272–276.
30. Weber M, Bissot T, Servet E, et al. A high-protein, high-fiber diet designed for weight loss improves satiety in dogs. *J Vet Intern Med*, 2007; 21(6):1203–1208.
31. Prola L, Dobenecker B, Mussa PP, Kienzle E. Influence of cellulose fibre length on faecal quality, mineral excretion and nutrient digestibility in cat. *J Anim Physiol Anim Nutr (Berl)*, 2010; 94(3):362–367.
32. de Haan V, Istasse L, Jakovljevic S, et al. Effects of cellulose, pectin and guar gum on gastric emptying, digestibility and absorption in resting dogs. *Proc Nutr Soc*, 1990; 49:146A.
33. Isaksson G, Lundquist I, Ihse I. Effect of dietary fiber on pancreatic enzyme activity in vitro. *Gastroenterology*, 1982; 82:918–924.
34. Dikeman CL, Fahey GC. Viscosity as related to dietary fiber: a review. *Crit Rev Food Sci Nutr*, 2006; 46(8):649–663.
35. Li S, Guerine-Deremaux L., Pochat M, et al. NUTRIOSE dietary fiber supplementation improves insulin resistance and determinants of metabolic syndrome in overweight men: a double-blind, randomized, placebo-controlled study. *Appl Physiol Nutr Metab*, 2010; 35(6):773–782.
36. Lee SC, Prosky L, De Vries JW. Determination of total, soluble, and insoluble dietary fiber in foods: enzymatic-gravimetric method, MES-TRIS buffer; Collaborative study. *J AOAC Int*, 1992; 75:395–416.
37. Forbes GB. Lean body mass-body fat interrelationships in humans. *Nutr Rev*, 1987; 45(8):225–231.
38. Forbes GB. Body fat content influences the body composition response to nutrition and exercise. *Ann N Y Acad Sci*, 2000; 904:359–365.
39. Jewell DE, Toll PW. Canine protein requirement and circulating glucose concentration during weight loss. *FASEB J*, 2007. 21(6):A743.
40. Johnson HL, VanLoan MD, Belko AZ, et al. Changes in human body composition during calorie restriction with two levels of protein. *Nutr Res*, 1993; 13(4):407–415.
41. Halton TL, Hu FB. The effects of high protein diets on thermogenesis, satiety and weight loss: a critical review. *J Am Coll Nutr*, 2004; 23(5):373–385.
42. Vasconcellos RS, Borges NC, Goncalves KN, et al. Protein intake during weight loss influences the energy required for weight loss and maintenance in cats. *J Nutr*, 2009; 139(5):855–860.
43. Wei A, Fascetti AJ, Liu KJ, et al. Influence of a high-protein diet on energy balance in obese cats allowed ad libitum access to food. *J Anim Physiol Anim Nutr (Berl)*, 2011; 95(3):359–367.
44. Laflamme DP, Hannah SS. Increased dietary protein promotes fat loss and reduces loss of lean body mass during weight loss in cats. *Int J Appl Res Vet Med*, 2005; 3(2):62–68.

45. Jeusette I, Compagnucci M, Romano V, et al. Effects of high-protein or high-carbohydrate diets on weight loss in obese dogs. *Comp Cont Ed Pract Vet*, 2006; 28(Suppl 4A):69.

46. Hannah SS, Laflamme DP. Increased dietary protein spares lean body mass during weight loss in dogs. *J Vet Int Med*, 1998; 12:224.

47. Yamka RM, Frantz NZ, Friesen KG. Effects of 3 canine weight loss foods on body composition and obesity markers. *Intern J Appl Res Vet Med*, 2007; 5(3):125–132.

48. Zoran DL, Buffington CA. Effects of nutrition choices and lifestyle changes on the well-being of cats, a carnivore that has moved indoors. *J Am Vet Med Assoc*, 2011; 239(5):596–606.

49. Zoran DL. The carnivore connection to nutrition in cats. *J Am Vet Med Assoc*, 2002; 221(11):1559–1567.

50. Hewson-Hughes AK, Hewson-Hughes VL, Miller AT, et al. Geometric analysis of macronutrient selection in the adult domestic cat, *Felis catus*. *J Exp Biol*, 2011; 214(Pt 6):1039–1051.

51. Stanhope KL, Keim NL, Griffen SC, et al. Consumption of a low glycemic index diet containing fructose increases risk factors for metabolic disease while a high glycemic index diet containing glucose does not. *Conference 69th Annual Meeting of the American-Diabetes-Association*, June 2009; vol. 58.

52. Flickinger EA, Sunvold GD. Early nutritional management to reduce the risks of diabetes and obesity. *Canine Pediatric Symposium*, World Small Animal Veterinary Association, Mexico, 2005.

53. Nguyen P, Dumon H, Biourge V, Pouteau E. Glycemic and insulinemic responses after ingestion of commercial foods in healthy dogs: Influence of food composition. *J Nutr*, 1998; 128(12):2654S–2658S.

54. Bouchard GF, Sunvold GD. Effect of dietary carbohydrate source on postprandial plasma glucose and insulin concentration in cats. In: *Recent advances in canine and feline nutrition*. Iams Nutrition Symposium Proceedings. Wilmington, OH, 2000. Orange Frazer Press, pp. 91–102.

55. Swarbrick MM, Stanhope KL, Elliott SS, et al. Consumption of fructose-sweetened beverages for 10 weeks increases postprandial triacylglycerol and apolipoprotein-B concentrations in overweight and obese women. *Br J Nutr*, 2008; 100(5):947–952.

56. Stanhope KL, Schwarz JM, Keim NL, et al. Consuming fructose-sweetened, not glucose-sweetened, beverages increases visceral adiposity and lipids and decreases insulin sensitivity in overweight/obese humans. *J Clin Invest*, 2009; 119(5):1322–1334.

57. Roudebush P, Schoenherr WD, Delaney SJ. An evidence-based review of the use of nutraceuticals and dietary supplementation for the management of obese and overweight pets. *J Am Vet Med Assoc*, 2008; 232(11):1646–1655.

58. Blanchard G, Paragon BM, Milliat F, Lutton C. Dietary L-carnitine supplementation in obese cats alters carnitine metabolism and decreases ketosis during fasting and induced hepatic lipidosis. *J Nutr*, 2002; 132(2):204–210.

59. Saldanha Aoki M, Rodriguez Amaral Almeida AL, Navarro F, et al. Carnitine supplementation fails to maximize fat mass loss induced by endurance training in rats. *Ann Nutr Metab*, 2004; 48:90-94.

60. Brandsch C, Eder K. Effect of L-carnitine on weight loss and body composition of rats fed a hypocaloric diet. *Ann Nutr Metab*, 2002; 46(5):205–210.

61. Pan Y, Tavazzi I, Oberson JM, et al. Effects of isoflavones, CLA and L-carnitine on weight loss and oxidative stress in overweight dogs. *Comp Cont Ed Pract Vet*, 2008; 30(Suppl 3A):69 (Abstr.).

62. Allison DB, Fontaine KR, Heshka S, et al. Alternative treatments for weight loss: a critical review. *Crit Rev Food Sci Nutr*, 2001; 41(1):1–28.

63. Scarpace PJ, Kumar MV, Bouchard GF, et al. Dietary vitamin A supplementation: role in obesity and leptin regulation in the dog and cat. In: Reinhart GA, Carey DP (eds.). *Recent advances in canine and feline nutrition*. Vol III. Wilmington, Ohio: Orange Frazer Press, 2000; pp. 103–111.

64. Wang YW, Jones PJ. Conjugated linoleic acid and obesity control: efficacy and mechanisms. *Int J Obes Relat Metab Disord*, 2004; 28(8):941–955.
65. Azain MJ. Conjugated linoleic acid and its effects on animal products and health in single-stomached animals. *Proc Nutr Soc*, 2003; 62(2):319–328.
66. Bauer JE, Nagaoka D, Porterpan B, et al. Postprandial lipolytic activities, lipids, and carbohydrate metabolism are altered in dogs fed diacylglycerol meals containing high- and low-glycemic-index starches. *J Nutr*, 2006; 136:1955S–1957S.
67. Umeda T, Bauer JE, Otsuji K. Weight loss effect of dietary diacylglycerol in obese dogs. *J Anim Physiol Anim Nutr (Berl)*, 2006; 90(5–6):208–215.
68. Reglamento de Ejecución (UE) 2015/662 de la Comisión, de 28 de abril de 2015, relativo a la autorización de la L-carnitina y del L-tartrato de L-carnitina como aditivos en piensos para todas las especies animales.

Chapter 6. Dietary management in weight-loss programmes

1. Valtolina C, Favier RP. Feline Hepatic Lipidosis. Vet Clin North Am Small Anim Pract, 2017 May; 47(3):683–702.
2. Saker KE, Remillard RL. Chapter 25: Critical care nutrition and enteral-assisted feeding. In: Hand MS, Thatcher CD, Remillard RL, et al. (eds.). *Small Animal Clinical Nutrition*, 5th Edition. Topeka, Kansas: Mark Morris Institute, 2010; pp. 439–476.
3. Berg JM, Tymoczko JL, Stryer L. Food intake and starvation induce metabolic changes (Section 30.3). Synthesizing the molecules of life (Part III). In: *Biochemistry*, 5th edition, New York: W H Freeman, 2002.
4. Makhija S, Baker J. The subjective global assessment: a review of its use in clinical practice. *Nutr Clin Pract*, 2008; 23(4):405–409.
5. Fascetti AJ, Mauldin GE, Mauldin GN. Correlation between serum creatine kinase activities and anorexia in cats. *J Vet Intern Med*, 1997; 11(1):9–13.
6. Simon JC, Saker KE, Thomas E. Sensitivity of specific immune function tests to acute nutrient deprivation as indicators of nutritional status in a feline model. *Nutr Res*, 2000; 20(1):79–89.
7. Zoran DL. The carnivore connection to nutrition in cats. *J Am Vet Med Assoc*, 2002 Dec 1; 221(11):1559–1567.
8. Forbes GB. Lean body mass-body fat interrelationships in humans. *Nutr Rev*, 1987; 45(8):225–231.
9. Cava E, Yeat NC, Mittendorfer B. Preserving healthy muscle during weight loss. *Adv Nutr*, 2017 May 15; 8(3):511–519.
10. Pasanisi F, Contaldo F, de Simone G, Mancini M. Benefits of sustained moderate weight loss in obesity. *Nutr Metab Cardiovasc Dis*, 2001 Dec; 11(6):401–406.
11. Crowell-Davis SL, Barry K, Ballam JM, Laflamme DP. The effect of caloric restriction on the behavior of pen-housed dogs: transition from unrestricted to restricted diet; and The effect of caloric restriction on the behavior of pen-housed dogs: transition from restriction to maintenance diets and long-term effects. *Appl Anim Behav Sci*, 1995; 43(1):27–61.
12. Flanagan J, Bissot T, Hours MA, et al. Success of a weight loss plan for overweight dogs: the results of an international weight loss study. *PLoS One*, 2017 Sep 8; 12(9):184–199.
13. Jeusette I, Biourge V, Nguyen P, et al. Energy restriction during a weight loss program must be stricter in female than male dogs. Proceedings of the American College of Veterinary Internal Medicine. ACVIM Forum 2004, June. http://hdl.handle.net/2268/200011
14. Butterwick RF, Hawthorne AJ. Advances in dietary management of obesity in dogs and cats. *J Nutr*, 1998; 128:2771S–2775S.
15. Diez M, Nguyen P, Jeusette I, et al. Weight loss in obese dogs: evaluation of a high-protein, low-carbohydrate diet. *J Nutr*, 2002; 132:1685S–1687S.
16. Laflamme DP, Hannah SS. Increased dietary protein promotes fat loss and reduces loss of lean body mass during weight loss in cats. *Intern J Appl Res Vet Med*, 2005; 3(2):62–68.

17. German AJ, Holden SL, Bissot T, et al. Dietary energy restriction and successful weight loss in obese client-owned dogs. *J Vet Intern Med*, 2007; 21(6):1174–1180.
18. National Research Council (NRC). Subcommittee on Dog and Cat Nutrition, Committee on Animal Nutrition. *Nutrient Requirements of Dogs and Cats*. Washington, DC: The National Academies Press, 2006.
19. Elices-Minguez R. Energy requirements; How are energy requirements determined?; How is the energy contained in a food determined? In: *Practical atlas of nutrition and feeding in cats and dogs* Volume I. Zaragoza, Spain: Servet Editorial, 2017; pp. 18–21/70–71.
20. Finke MD. Evaluation of the energy requirements of adult kennel dogs. *J Nutr*, 1991; 121:S22–S28.
21. Finke MD, Lutschaunig MT. Energy requirements of adult Abyssinian cats. *Vet Clin Nutr*, 1995; 2:64.
22. Laflamme DP, Jackson JR. Weight loss protocols for overweight cats (abstract). *Vet Clin Nutr*, 1995; 2:143.
23. Wishnofsky M. Caloric equivalents of gained or lost weight. *Am J Clin Nutr*, 1958; 6(5):542-546.
24. McArdle WD, Katch FI, Katch VL. *Exercise physiology: energy, nutrition, and human performance*. 4th edition. Baltimore: Williams & Wilkins; 1996.
25. Butterwick RF, Markwell PJ. Changes in the body composition of cats during weight reduction by controlled dietary energy restriction. *Vet Rec*, 1996 Apr 13; 138(15):354–357.

Chapter 7. Treatment of obesity

1. Roudebush P, Schoenherr WD, Delaney SJ. An evidence-based review of the use of therapeutic foods, owner education, exercise, and drugs for the management of obese and overweight pets. *J Am Vet Med Assoc*, 2008 Sep 1; 233(5):717–725.
2. Elices-Minguez R. Other methods to evaluate the energy in foods. In: *Practical atlas of nutrition and feeding in cats and dogs* Volume I. Zaragoza, Spain: Servet Editorial, 2017; pp. 72–73.
3. White GA, Ward L, Pink C, et al. "Who's been a good dog?" – owner perceptions and motivations for treat giving. *Prev Vet Med*, 2016; 132:14–19.
4. Downes MJ, Devitt C, Downes MT, More SJ. Understanding the context for pet cat and dog feeding and exercising behaviour among pet owners in Ireland: a qualitative study. *Ir Vet J*, 2017; 70:29.
5. Robertson ID. The association of exercise, diet and other factors with owner-perceived obesity in privately owned dogs from metropolitan Perth, WA. *Prev Vet Med*, 2003 Apr 30; 58(1–2):75–83.
6. Courcier EA, Thomson RM, Mellor DJ, Yam PS. An epidemiological study of environmental factors associated with canine obesity. *J Small Anim Pract*, 2010 Jul; 51(7):362–367.
7. Kienzle E, Bergler R, Mandernach A. A comparison of the feeding behavior and the human-animal relationship in owners of normal and obese dogs. *J Nutr*, 1998; 128:2779S–27782S.
8. Laflamme DP, Abood SK, Fascetti AJ, et al. Pet feeding practices of dog and cat owners in the United States and Australia. *J Am Vet Med Assoc*, 2008 Mar 1; 232(5):687–694.
9. Jericó M, Silva A, Pereira V, Tirapelli A. Effects of diet and physical activity in the clinical evaluation of obese dogs. *World Small Animal Veterinary Association World Congress Proceedings*, 2006.
10. National Research Council (NRC). Subcommittee on Dog and Cat Nutrition, Committee on Animal Nutrition. Physical activity and environment, chapter 11. *Nutrient Requirements of Dogs and Cats*. Washington, DC: The National Academies Press, 2006.
11. Vitger AD, Stallknecht BM, Nielsen DH, Bjornvad CR. Integration of a physical training program in a weight loss plan for overweight pet dogs. *J Am Vet Med Assoc*, 2016 Jan 15; 248(2):174–182.
12. Elices-Minguez R. How much energy does a dog spend when running?; Other system changes in aginng. In: *Practical atlas of nutrition and feeding in cats and dogs* Volume II. Zaragoza, Spain: Servet Editorial, 2017; pp. 68-69/48-49.

13. Lund EM, Armstrong PJ, Kirk CA, Klausner JS. Prevalence and risk factors for obesity in adult dogs from private US veterinary practices. *Int J Appl Res Vet Med*, 2006; 4(2):177–186.

14. Case LP, Carey DP, Hirakawa DA, et al. Obesity. In: Case LP, Carey DP, Hirakawa DA, et al. (eds.). *Canine and feline nutrition*. 3rd ed. St Louis: Mosby Inc, 2011; pp. 313–342.

15. Pedersen BK, Febbraio MA. Muscles, exercise and obesity: skeletal muscle as a secretory organ. *Nat Rev Endocrinol*, 2012 Apr 3; 8(8):457–465.

16. Kanzleiter T, Rath M, Görgens SW, et al. The myokine decorin is regulated by contraction and involved in muscle hypertrophy. *Biochem Biophys Res Commun*, 2014 Jul 25; 450(2):1089–1094.

17. Boström P, Wu J, Jedrychowski MP, et al. A PGC1-α-dependent myokine that drives brown-fat-like development of white fat and thermogenesis. *Nature*, 2012 Jan 11; 481(7382):463–468.

18. You T, Arsenis NC, Disanzo BL, Lamonte MJ. Effects of exercise training on chronic inflammation in obesity: current evidence and potential mechanisms. *Sports Med*, 2013 Apr; 43(4):243–256.

19. Kienzle E, Bergler R. Human-animal relationship of owners of normal and overweight cats. *J Nutr*, 2006 Jul; 136(7 Suppl):1947S–1950S.

20. Kushner RF, Blatner DJ, Jewell DE, Rudloff K. The PPET study: people and pets exercising together. *Obesity (Silver Spring)*, 2006 Oct; 14(10):1762–1770.

21. Jewell DE, Rudloff K, Kushner RF. People and pets exercising together. A comparison of the effect of a canine weight loss program to a combined dog/owner weight loss program (abstr), in: *Proceedings. North American Association for the Study of Obesity*, 2004: 251-P.

22. Wren JA, Gossellin J, Sunderland SJ. Dirlotapide: a review of its properties and role in the management of obesity in dogs. *J Vet Pharmacol Ther*, 2007 Aug; 30 Suppl 1:11–16.

23. European Medicine Agency. *Yarvitan. Summary of Product Characteristics*. Janssen Animal Health, 2006; B-2340 Beerse, Belgium. Available at: http://www.ema.europa.eu/ema/index.jsp?curl=pages/medicines/veterinary/medicines/000113/vet_med_000196.jsp.

24. European Medicine Agency. *Xenical, INN-Orlistat.* http://www.ema.europa.eu/docs/en_GB/document_library/EPAR_-_Scientific_Discussion/human/000154/WC500058424.pdf.

25. Pi-Sunyer X, Astrup A, Fujioka K, et al. A randomized, controlled trial of 3.0 mg of liraglutide in weight management. *N Engl J Med*, July 2015; 373(1):11–22.

26. Gilor C, Graves TK, Gilor S, et al. The GLP-1 mimetic exenatide potentiates insulin secretion in healthy cats. *Domest Anim Endocrinol*, 2011 Jul; 41(1):42–49.

27. Hall MJ, Adin CA, Borin-Crivellenti S, et al. Pharmacokinetics and pharmacodynamics of the glucagon-like peptide-1 analog liraglutide in healthy cats. *Domest Anim Endocrinol*, 2015 Apr; 51:114–121.

28. Richey JM, Woolcott OO, Stefanovski D, et al. Rimonabant prevents additional accumulation of visceral and subcutaneous fat during high-fat feeding in dogs. *Am J Physiol Endocrinol Metab*, 2009 Jun; 296(6):E1311–E1318.

29. Smith SR, Weissman NJ, Anderson CM, et al. Multicenter, placebo-controlled trial of lorcaserin for weight management. *N Engl J Med*, 2010 Jul 15; 363(3):245–56. doi: 10.1056/NEJMoa0909809.

30. Gustafson A, king C, Rey JA. Lorcaserin (Belviq) a selective serotonin 5-HT2C agonist in the treatment of obesity. *P T*, 2013 Sep; 38(9):525–534.

31. Xu J, Dz Chen J. Effects of sibutramine on gastric emptying, intestinal motility and rectal tone in dogs. *Dig Dis Sci*, 2008 Jan; 53(1):155–162.

32. Plumb DC. *Plumb's veterinary drug handbook*. 9th edition. Wiley-Blackwell, 2018.

33. Peterson KL, Lee JA, Hovda LR. Phenylpropanolamine toxicosis in dogs: 170 cases (2004-2009). *J Am Vet Med Assoc*, 2011 Dec 1; 239(11):1463–1469.

34. Sherman MM, Ungureanu S, Rey JA. Naltrexone/bupropion ER (Contrave) newly approved treatment option for chronic weight management in obese adults. *P T*, 2016 Mar; 41(3):164–172.
35. Paganelli MO, Tanus-Santos JE, Sabha M, et al. Hemodynamic effects of bupropion in anesthetized dogs. *Eur J Pharmacol*, 2006 Jan 13; 530(1–2):124–127.
36. Faria GFR. A brief history of bariatric surgery. *Porto Biomed J*, 2017; 2(3):90–92.
37. Buchwald H, Avidor Y, Braunwald E, et al. Bariatric surgery: a systematic review and meta-analysis. *JAMA*, 2004 Oct 13; 292(14):1724–1737.
38. Monkhouse SJ, Morgan JD, Norton SA. Complications of bariatric surgery: presentation and emergency management–a review. *Ann R Coll Surg Engl*, 2009 May; 91(4):280–286.
39. Rao RS, Rao V, Kini S. Animal models in bariatric surgery--a review of the surgical techniques and postsurgical physiology. *Obes Surg*, 2010 Sep; 20(9):1293–1305.
40. Hunt GB, Wong J, Kuan S. Liposuction for removal of lipomas in 20 dogs. *J Small Anim Pract*, 2011 Aug; 52(8):419–425.
41. Böttcher P, Klüter S, Krastel D, Grevel V. Liposuction-removal of giant lipomas for weight loss in a dog with severe hip osteoarthritis. *J Small Anim Pract*, 2007 Jan; 48(1):46–48.

Chapter 8. Prevention of obesity

1. Wing RR, Hill JO. Successful weight loss maintenance. *Annu Rev Nutr*, 2001; 21:323–341.
2. Wing RR, Phelan S. Long-term weight loss maintenance. *Am J Clin Nutr*, 2005; 82(1 Suppl):222S–225S.
3. MacLean PS, Higgins JA, Jackman MR, et al. Peripheral metabolic responses to prolonged weight reduction that promote rapid, efficient regain in obesity-prone rats. *Am J Physiol Regul Integr Comp Physiol*, 2006; 290(6):R1577–R1588.
4. MacLean PS, Higgins JA, Johnson GC, et al. Enhanced metabolic efficiency contributes to weight regain after weight loss in obesity-prone rats. *Am J Physiol Regul Integr Comp Physiol*, 2004; 287(6):R1306–R1315.
5. MacLean PS, Higgins JA, Johnson GC, et al. Metabolic adjustments with the development, treatment, and recurrence of obesity in obesity-prone rats. *Am J Physiol Regul Integr Comp Physiol*, 2004; 287(2):R288–R297.
6. Weiss EC, Galuska DA, Kettel Khan L, et al. Weight regain in U.S. adults who experienced substantial weight loss, 1999-2002. *Am J Prev Med*, 2007; 33(1):34–40.
7. Ilagan J, Bhutani V, Archer P, et al. Estimation of body composition changes during weight cycling by bioelectrical impedance analysis in rats. *J Appl Physiol*, 1993; 74(5):2092–2098.
8. Kochan Z, Karbowska J, Swierczynski J. The effects of weight cycling on serum leptin levels and lipogenic enzyme activities in adipose tissue. *J Physiol Pharmacol*, 2006; 57(Suppl 6):115–127.
9. Nagaoka D, Mitsuhashi Y, Angell R, et al. Re-induction of obese body weight occurs more rapidly and at lower caloric intake in beagles. *J Anim Physiol Anim Nutr (Berl)*, 2010 Jun; 94(3):287–292.
10. Mugford RA. External influences on feeding of carnivores. In: Kare MR, Maller O (eds.). *The Chemical Senses and Nutrition*. New York: Academic Press, 1977; pp. 25–50.
11. National Research Council (NRC). Subcommittee on Dog and Cat Nutrition, Committee on Animal Nutrition. *Nutrient Requirements of Dogs and Cats*. Washington, DC: The National Academies Press, 2006.
12. Sumithran P, Prendergast LA, Delbridge E, et al. Long-term persistence of hormonal adaptations to weight loss. *N Engl J Med*, 2011 Oct 27; 365(17):1597–1604.
13. Aller EE, Larsen TM, Claus H, et al. Weight loss maintenance in overweight subjects on ad libitum diets with high or low protein content and glycemic index: The DIOGENES trial 12-month results. *Int J Obes (Lond)*, 2014; 38:1511–1517.

14. Muhammad HFL, Vink RG, Roumans NJT, et al. Dietary intake after weight loss and the risk of weight regain: macronutrient composition and inflammatory properties of the diet. *Nutrients*, 2017 Nov 2; 9(11):1205.
15. Thaiss CA, Itav S, Rothschild D., et al. Persistent microbiome alterations modulate the rate of post-dieting weight regain. *Nature*, 2016; 540:544–551.
16. Greenway FL. Physiological adaptations to weight loss and factors favouring weight regain. *Int J Obes (Lond)*, 2015 Aug; 39(8):1188-1196.
17. Anderson JW, Konz EC, Frederich RC, Wood CL. Long-term weight-loss maintenance: a meta-analysis of US studies. *Am J Clin Nutr*, 2001; 74(5):579–584.
18. Grief SN, Miranda RL. Weight loss maintenance. *Am Fam Physician*, 2010 Sep 15; 82(6):630–634.
19. Voils CI, Olsen MK, Gierisch JM, et al. Maintenance of weight loss after initiation of nutrition training: a randomized trial. *Ann Intern Med*, 2017 Apr 4; 166(7):463–471.
20. Kwon HN, Nam SS, Park YK. Effect on 12-week intensive dietary and exercise program on weight reduction and maintenance in obese women with weight cycling history. *Clin Nutr Res*, 2017 Jul; 6(3):183–197.
21. Wing RR, Tate DF, Gorin AA, et al. A self-regulation program for maintenance of weight loss. *N Engl J Med*, 2006; 355(15):1563–1571.
22. Dulloo AG, Montani JP. Pathways from dieting to weight regain, to obesity and to the metabolic syndrome: an overview. *Obes Rev*, 2015 Feb; 16(Suppl 1):1–6.
23. Svetkey LP, Stevens VJ, Brantley PJ, et al. Comparison of strategies for sustaining weight loss: the Weight Loss Maintenance randomized controlled trial. *JAMA*, 2008; 299(10):1139–1148.
24. Ryder JR, Gross AC, Fox CK, et al. Factors associated with long-term weight-loss maintenance following bariatric surgery in adolescents with severe obesity. *Int J Obes (Lond)*, 2018 Jan; 42(1):102–107.
25. Chin SO, Keum C, Woo J, et al. Successful weight reduction and maintenance by using a smartphone application in those with overweight and obesity. *Sci Rep*, 2016 Nov 7; 6:345–363.
26. Divol G, Priymenko N. A new model for evaluating maintenance energy requirements in dogs: allometric equation from 319 pet dogs. *J Nutr Sci*, 2017; 6:e53.
27. Connor MM, Labato MA, Laflamme DP. Variation in maintenance energy requirements of pet dogs. *Purina Nutrition Forum Proceedings Supplement to Compendium of Continuing Education for the Practicing Veterinarian*, 2000; 23(9a):84.
28. Mullis RA, Witzel AL, Price J. Maintenance energy requirements of odor detection, explosive detection and human detection working dogs. *PeerJ*, 2015 Feb 24; 3:e767.
29. Elices-Minguez R. Weight gain in puppies and kittens; Requirements during growth. In: *Practical atlas of nutrition and feeding in cats and dogs* Volume II. Zaragoza, Spain: Servet Editorial, 2017; pp. 30–31, 36–39.